ORTHOPATHIC MEDICINE

The Unification of Orthopedics with Osteopathy
Through the Fascial Distortion Model

Third Edition

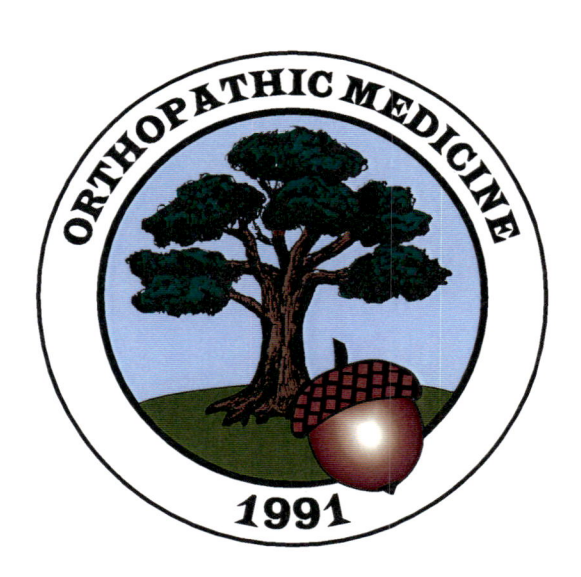

Stephen Typaldos, D.O.

Illustrations by Anita Crane

First Edition 1997
Second Edition 1998
Third Edition 1999

All rights reserved. No part of this publication may be reproduced, stored in a retrieval system, or transmitted in any form or by any means, electronic or mechanical, photocopying, recording, or otherwise, without the prior written permission of the author.

This book is not intended as a substitute for the medical advice of a physician. Shown in this text are possible considerations and treatments for patients with injuries or medical conditions. It is the responsibility of the treating physician, relying on his/her experience and knowledge, to determine the best course of therapy for each patient. Each physician is cautioned to use his or her best judgment before employing these or any other treatment modalities. The good clinician will modify the treatments according to the special needs of each individual patient. The author and publisher cannot be responsible for any clinical decisions made by the practitioner, or the side effects or adverse outcomes of any particular treatment discussed in this book.

©Stephen Typaldos, D.O., 1997, 1998, 1999

ISBN 0-9659641-2-4

FOREWORD TO PHYSICIANS

Orthopathic medicine: What is it? What can it do?

You are holding in your hands a road map that guides you into a new era of treating orthopedic and structural injuries. Much more than just a collection of manipulative techniques, orthopathic medicine is a distinct system of diagnosing and treating based on a completely new model of medical thought. Here are two clinical examples that illustrate how the understanding of fascial pathology has impacted my patients:

> An 18 year old male came limping into the office after spraining his ankle. The fact that he walked with a limp and could not run was not a trifling concern to him. As a local star soccer player he had been invited to try out for a spot on the state team so he needed to be able to perform his skills at a high level — immediately. Therefore he was treated orthopathically, meaning that specific physical alterations of the fascia around the ankle were identified and corrected. Following the treatment he ran without pain. The next day he attended the tryout and made the team.

> For the past five years, a 32 year old woman complained of bilateral frozen shoulders with progressively worsening pain. At home she was unable to brush her hair and could barely raise her hand to her mouth. Although her orthopedist recommended an operation, she refused because of her fear of surgery. On first exam in my office, her abduction was limited to 45° bilaterally. Following the first treatment in which I used my hands to smooth out the wrinkled fascia, 90% of the pain was relieved and abduction improved to 140°. After two more sessions she was pain-free and both shoulders exhibited normal range of motion.

These clinical results are the power that fuels orthopathy. The door is now open for us all, and the potential is just starting to be realized.

Dr. Typaldos' book gives us a better grip on the tail of the squirrel. So read on, and welcome to orthopathic medicine!

Brian Knight, D.O.
Assistant Director
Osteopathic Manipulative Medicine Dept.
Eastmoreland Hospital
Portland, Oregon
U.S.A.

This book is dedicated to all the physicians, surgeons, and osteopaths around the world who practice orthopathic medicine.

ABOUT THE BOOK / ACKNOWLEDGEMENTS

The first writings for *Orthopathic Medicine: The Unification of Orthopedics with Osteopathy Through the Fascial Distortion Model* were begun on a snowy Maine winter day in January 1996. It was almost twelve months later and a half a world away that the prototype edition became the first teaching text for orthopathy (printed in English for the students at Wiener Schule für Osteopathie). Now three years (one Japanese and two English editions) later, this third edition (soon to be in German and French) becomes the most updated and upgraded book on orthopathic medicine ever published.

This new edition of *Orthopathic Medicine* is physically divided into four separate sections, each of which has a distinct function and presents material in its own format:

    Section One: Introduction to Theory and Techniques
    Section Two: Treatment of Specific Conditions
    Section Three: Case Histories
    Section Four: Addendum

Section One is where general fascial distortion model concepts and techniques are explained. Section Two is the nuts and bolts of how to treat actual injuries such as sore shoulders and sprained ankles. Section Three gives case histories with discussions that challenge the reader intellectually, and clinically demonstrate how injuries and conditions are envisioned and treated orthopathically. Section Four contains quick references to terms, techniques, distortion types, and the glossary — which many physicians feel is the most frequently accessed part of the book.

A number of individuals have contributed to the process of creating this book:
    Anita Crane (artist): Her three years of drawings for this book include collages, clay models, computer enhancements, and a wide assortment of creative and artistic processes to visually enhance the orthopathic concepts and techniques.
    Marjorie Kasten (chief editor, Orthopathic Global Health Publications, OGHP): Executor of the literally thousands of processes that result in a book: editing, grammar, typing, transcribing, computer manipulations, layout, photos, correspondence, problem checker, problem solver, content critic, and orthopathic physical therapist.
    John Kasten (associate editor, OGHP): Sentence structure and grammar specialist.
    Irv Marsters (printer of the English texts): This high quality book which you are holding in your hands, was physically produced at his Bangor Letter Shop.

Barrie Oldham (editor of the Orthopathic Medicine Webpage): Strongest supporter of orthopathy through its infancy, and still its leading advocate.

Koichi Hiratsuka (publisher, Sky East): Brought orthopathic medicine to Japan through the seminars and the Japanese edition of the book.

Eric Wühr (publisher, Verlag für Ganzheltliche Medicin, VGM): Produced the German edition of *Orthopathic Medicine*.

Many others to thank are my colleagues and friends from around the world who have supported orthopathy. In particular my appreciation is extended to Raphael van Assche and Raimund Engel at the Wiener Schule für Osteopathie, Louis Rommeveaux and Patrick Feval at the College International D'Osteopathie, and Angelo Lucas of the Associação E Registo Dos Osteopatas De Portugal. Also, I'd like to acknowledge my five assistants: Rob Truax, Nori Onishi, Barrie Oldham, Georg Harrer, and Patrice Castelain, who have helped teach seminars in Austria, France, Portugal, Japan, and the United States.

Not to be forgotten are the contributions of my patients both current and past, who have volunteered for (and perhaps endured) each of the new and developing treatments. And finally, I'd like to thank my family for supporting me through these long months of writing, teaching, and traveling.

Stephen Typaldos, D.O.
Bangor, Maine
U.S.A.

Contents

Section One: Introduction To Theory and Techniques

Chapter   **Page**

1. Introduction 3
2. Principal Types of Fascial Distortions 12
3. Triggerbands and Triggerband Technique 17
4. Herniated Triggerpoints and Herniated Triggerpoint Therapy 25
5. Continuum Distortions and Continuum Technique 29
6. Folding Distortions and Folding Technique 35
7. Cylinder Distortions and Cylinder Technique 45
8. Tectonic Fixations and Tectonic Technique 51
9. Synopsis of Selected Fascial Distortion Concepts 59

Section Two: Treatment of Specific Conditions

10. The Orthopathic Treatment of Cervical, Thoracic, and Lumbar Strains 75
11. The Orthopathic Treatment of the Sore Shoulder 89
12. The Orthopathic Treatment of Ankle Sprains 111
13. Fascial Distortion Techniques in the Emergency Room 127
14. The Orthopathic Approach to Treating Post-Stroke Spastic Paralysis 145

Section Three: Case Histories

1. Ankle Pain in a 41 Year Old Man 153
2. Shoulder Pain in a 50 Year Old Woman 155
3. Low Back Pain in a 46 Year Old Man 157
4. Osteoarthritic Knee Pain in a 71 Year Old Woman 161
5. Heel Pain in an 11 Year Old Boy 163
6. Upper Arm Pain Following Flu Shot 165
7. Low Back Pain in a Woman with Multiple Compression Fractures 165
8. Fibromyalgia in a 45 Year Old Woman 167
9. Sprained Ankle in a 26 Year Old Woman 169
10. Upper Arm Pain in a 67 Year Old Man 171
11. Shoulder Pain in a 42 Year Old Woman 173
12. Chest Wall Pain in a 25 Year Old Man 175
13. Shoulder Pain in a 43 Year Old Woman 175
14. Post-Stroke Spastic Paralysis Patient 177
15. Upper Back Pain in a 21 Year Old Woman 179
16. Ankle Pain in a 39 Year Old Woman 181

17. Left Lower Extremity Weakness in a Woman with Post-Polio Syndrome 183
18. Frozen Shoulder/Reflex Sympathetic Dystrophy-Like Symptoms
    in a 38 Year Old Woman 185
19. Frozen Shoulder in a 45 Year Old Woman 187
20. Spinal Stenosis in a 52 Year Old Man 189
21. Elbow Pain in a 57 Year Old Man 191
22. Ankle Pain in an 80 Year Old Woman 193
23. Acute Abdominal Pain in a 62 Year Old Woman 195
24. Psoriatic Arthritis in a 43 Year Old Woman 197

SECTION FOUR: ADDENDUM

Summary of Common Orthopathic Conditions, Body Language, and Treatments 201
Treatment of Combination Distortions 212
Orthopathic Abbreviations 213
Table of Principal Types of Fascial Distortions 214
Table of Triggerband Subtypes 216
Table of Herniated Triggerpoint Subtypes 217
Table of Continuum Distortion Subtypes 218
Table of Folding Distortion Subtypes 219
Table of Cylinder Distortion Subtypes 220
Glossary 221
Index 241
About the Author 248
Author's Postscript Note 249

FIGURES AND CHARTS

Hemiplegic Patient	5
Correction of a Pulled Muscle	7
Clothing as a Mechanical Sensory System	8
Cornstarch/Water Phenomenon	9
Fascial Bands	12
Zip Lock Analogy	18
Acute and Chronic Triggerbands	21
Triggerband Technique of the Anterior Shoulder Pathway	23
Herniated Triggerpoint Therapy of the SCHTP	26
Cows Through the Barn Door Analogy	27
Continuum Distortions and the Ice/Slush/Water Analogy	31
Treatment of Lateral Ankle Continuum Distortion	32
Unfolding Shoulder Injury and Treatment	36
Refolding Shoulder Injury and Treatment	38
Folding/Thrusting Manipulations of the Cervical Spine	40
Hallelujah Maneuver and Wall Technique	41
Chair Technique	42
Ball Therapy	43
Inversion Traction	44
Cylinder Distortion of Brachial Fascia	46
Treatment with Double Thumb Cylinder Technique	47
Schematics of Uninjured and Distorted Cylinder Fascia	48
Marching Down the Forearm with Indian Burn Cylinder Technique	48
Double Thumb Cylinder Technique for Deep and Superficial Layers of Cylinder Fascia	49
Squeegee Cylinder Technique of the Lower Leg	49
Double Thumb Compression Cylinder Variant of the Thigh	50
Tectonic Fixation of the Shoulder	52
Slow Tectonic Pump	53
Frogleg and Reverse Frogleg Manipulations of the Shoulder	54
Frogleg and Reverse Frogleg Manipulations of the Hip	56
Kirksville Crunch and Double Pisiform Thrust	57
Road Map Analogy and Forearm Fracture	60
Ligamental Triggerband	64
Achilles Tendon Tear	65
Erythema, Bruising, and Hemorrhagic Petechia	71
Treatment of Star Triggerband	76
Treatment of Upper Trapezius (Shoulder to Mastoid) Triggerband	76
Double Thumb Compression Cylinder Variant	78

Treatment of Posterior Shoulder Triggerband Pathway	80
Star Unfolding and First-Rib Refolding Manipulations	81
Low Back Pain Table	83
Body Language and Treatments for Low Back Pain	86
Sore Shoulder Body Language	90
Three Important Shoulder Motions	92
Subtle Shoulder Motions	93
Orthopathic Flow Chart of the Acutely Sore Shoulder	94
Orthopathic Flow Chart of the Chronically Sore Shoulder	95
Common Shoulder Triggerband Pathways and Treatments	106
Treatment of Supraclavicular Herniated Triggerpoint	107
Continuum Technique of the Shoulder	107
Folding Techniques of the Shoulder	108
Cylinder Techniques of the Upper Arm	109
Tectonic Techniques of the Shoulder	110
Three Types of Ankle Sprains	112
Comparing Ankle Sprain Types	113
Typical Swelling Patterns in Ankle Sprain Types	114
Ankle Sprains of All Three Types Demonstrate Decreased Dorsiflexion	115
Orthopathic Flow Chart of the Acutely Sprained Ankle	117
Continuum Technique of the Ankle	118
Triggerband Technique of the Lateral Ankle Pathway	121
Folding Technique of the Ankle	123
Body Language of Flank HTP and Flank Triggerband	137
Treatment of Flank HTP	138
Treatment of Flank Triggerband	138
Post-Stroke Spastic Paralysis Patient	146

SECTION ONE

INTRODUCTION TO THEORY AND TECHNIQUES

Chapter 1

INTRODUCTION

Orthopathic medicine is the branch of the healing arts, which through the fascial distortion model (FDM), integrates manipulative treatments into orthopedic practice. Within this model, alterations of the connecting structures of the musculoskeletal system (ligaments, tendons, fascial bands, retinacula, etc.) form during injury and are responsible for a wide range of conditions such as frozen shoulders and sprained ankles. The orthopathic approach adds not only a diagnostic dimension to the interpretation of the injury but a practical application as well. And since orthopathic manipulative (and in the future, surgical) treatments are specifically designed to correct fascial distortions, the results often surpass what either orthopedic or osteopathic philosophy deem possible. For instance, in the frozen shoulder discussed in Case History #11, excision of a portion of the clavicle was averted because of the competitiveness of the orthopathic treatment (restoration of function in two sessions). And in treating sprained ankles (see Case History #9) the expected outcome is an *immediate* alleviation of symptoms with normalization of motion and strength.

With orthopathy, each injury is anatomically envisioned through the FDM which conceptually bridges together subjective complaints (utilizing body language and the verbal description of discomfort), mechanism of injury, and objective findings to form an orthopathic diagnosis. Just as with the mathematical equation $a \times b = c$, if any two of the variables are known, the third can be deduced. Therefore when someone sprains an ankle from falling off a horse and has bi-malleolar swelling with pain deep in the joint, this means that the injury occurred from the foot becoming caught in the stirrup (real life example). The mechanism of injury (foot becoming pinned while the ankle is tractioned) becomes known because the symptoms and physical findings match only one of the principal fascial distortion types (folding). And once we know the mechanism of forces that caused the injury we can correct the anatomical distortion. Consequently, the best therapy for treating this sprained ankle is not the traditional R.I.C.E. (rest, ice, compression, and elevation) but instead modified traction manipulation.

Although physicians tend to automatically view musculoskeletal injuries orthopedically, when the accompanying fascial pathology is integrated within the diagnosis, a different appreciation of that same injury often results. In other words, the orthopathic diagnosis adds the precise manner in which the fascia is physically altered to the orthopedic interpretation. In the case of sprained ankles, for example, when listening to a large number of patients describe their symptoms, it can be noted that some talk about a sharp pain in the lateral ankle, while others complain of a pulling pain up the leg, and yet others mention a deep ache in the joint. Whereas in the orthopedic and osteopathic models the relevance of these various symptoms may seem unclear, this is not the case in orthopathy. In the FDM these descriptions signify that there are three types of sprained ankles, each with different symptoms, presentations, and mechanisms of injury.

In addition to offering radically new diagnostic interpretations and techniques, the FDM envisions other approaches from an anatomical perspective and can predict results of specific osteopathic and orthopedic therapies (such as the efficacy of thrusting manipulation in chronic pain and steroid injections for sore shoulders). And because the fascial distortion model emphasizes the sensory and mechanical function of fascia, orthopathic medicine is revolutionizing rehabilitative strategies for post-stroke spastic paralysis and other neuro/fascial conditions.

What distinguishes orthopathy from osteopathy and orthopedics is this philosophy: Before any manipulative techniques, surgical procedures, pharmaceutical agents, or physical therapy modalities are utilized, the anatomical consequences of those interventions are contemplated through the FDM. For instance, although the osteopathic goal of high-velocity low-amplitude manipulation (HVLA) of the neck is to improve joint mobility — what does this mean anatomically? Orthopathically, cervical HVLA:

1. Forces fixated facet joints to slide
2. Unfolds and untorques folding fascia
3. Refolds folding fascia which then unfolds in a less contorted way

Thus HVLA is a good choice for some injuries (i.e., folding distortions and tectonic fixations) but not for others (everted continuum distortions, cylinder distortions, herniated triggerpoints, or triggerbands with adhesions). The orthopathic approach is therefore able to assist the physician or surgeon in choosing, modifying, and developing specific techniques that correct underlying anatomical distortions.

THE FASCIAL DISTORTION MODEL

The fascial distortion model is the anatomical perspective in which virtually every musculoskeletal injury is envisioned as consisting of one or more of six distinct alterations in the body's fascia (see Chapter 2). Therefore, injuries as seemingly diverse as sprained ankles, frozen shoulders, and lumbar strains are clinically diagnosed and treated as location-specific variations of this common pathological theme.

Although the most obvious physical finding of any fascial distortion is loss of motion, each of the six types has clinical signature symptoms and presentations which, in the practice of orthopathic medicine, are matched to the corresponding corrective manipulative treatments. For the orthopathic osteopath or orthopedist the clinical approach to evaluating and treating a musculoskeletal injury typically follows this sequence:

1. History and physical examination (including laboratory and x-ray studies, if necessary)
2. Orthopedic diagnosis
3. Synthesis of body language with physical findings and description of symptoms to make the orthopathic diagnosis
4. Correction of the injury with the corresponding fascial distortion techniques

In treating simple acute injuries, only one FDM technique may be needed since clinically only one distortion type may be present. But in a more complicated or long-standing injury, several or all six distortions may occur and thus several or all six FDM techniques may be employed. For example, in a frozen shoulder secondary to post-stroke spastic paralysis, multitudes of distortions have formed which not only restrict motion but are indirectly responsible for the concurrent spasm, tremor, and hypertonia (see Chapter 14). The focus of the initial treatments is to correct each of the involved distortions *one by one* until the shoulder regains normal range of motion.

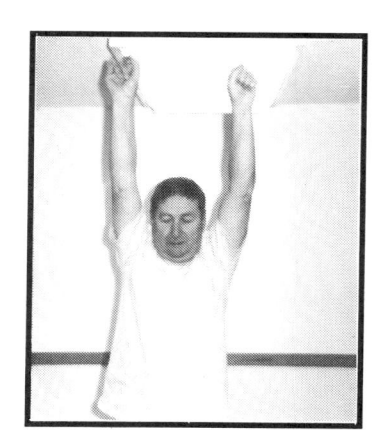

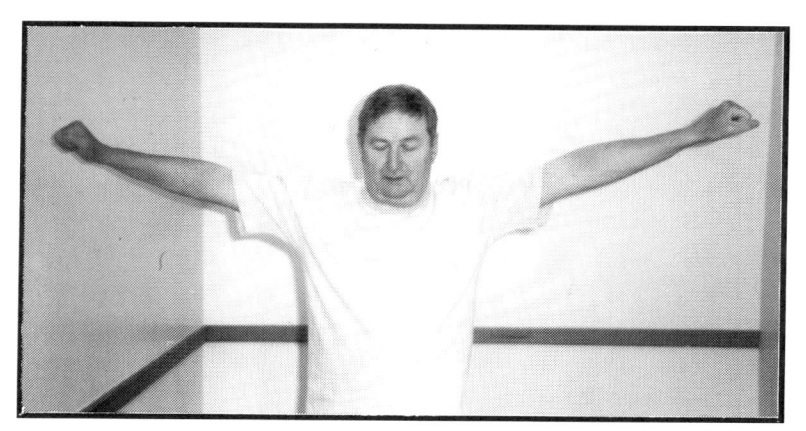

Figure 1-1. Hemiplegic patient two and a half years following stroke and six months after initiating orthopathic treatments, demonstrating improving function of previously frozen right shoulder and spastic right upper extremity

Since in orthopathy the traditional orthopedic diagnosis is often considered to be incomplete, FDM terminology is introduced to illustrate the differences in orthopedic and orthopathic perspectives. One specific example of this is a pulled muscle. In the orthopedic model, a pulled muscle is considered to be a tear in the muscle, whereas in the FDM it is viewed as a distorted fascial band (known as a triggerband) which has become stuck in the belly of the muscle. This difference in what the injury is called influences how it is envisioned, and therefore, how it is treated. The implication of the orthopedic concept of a pulled muscle is that the tissue has been traumatized and needs time to recover. But when looking at the same injury from the fascial distortion perspective, the treatment connotation of stuck fascial fibers is that they need to be *unstuck*.

The FDM concept of pulled muscles becomes possible because of the anatomical arrangement of fascial bands. Some bands near muscles have origins and insertions on either side of the muscle with a pathway that runs through the muscle. When the fascial band becomes injured (and thus distorted), it physically crumples and twists. Whenever the muscle surrounding the band subsequently contracts, the twisted fascial fibers act as a kink which impedes some of the contracting muscle fibers. This is clinically evident by a painful, weak, and poorly coordinated contraction.

Although the traditional approach of resting a pulled muscle empirically seems to be of benefit, it has a major drawback in the overall amount of time, pain, and disability before the symptoms abate. Fascial distortion treatments, in contrast, manually correct the distortion, which allows for an almost instantaneous treatment result with virtually no recuperative time, and little chance of recurrence.

Orthopathically the distorted band is corrected by manually forcing the twist through the belly of the muscle and untwisting the twisted fibers. Once this is done, the fascial band is no longer kinked and the muscle can glide around it each time it contracts. The corrected fibers not only result in the patient being asymptomatic, but also in the muscle once again exhibiting normal contractile strength.

In the conventional treatment of pulled muscles, the injury is rested or splinted, which leads to atrophy of the muscle and allows more room for the twist to work its way back out of the belly of the muscle. Exercising (another traditional treatment option) may also seem beneficial since repetitive contractions may force the twist out. The negative aspect of these approaches is that the anatomical distortion is still present and has not been corrected. The same injury is likely to occur again when the muscle forcefully contracts and the twist is pulled back into its belly. In the fascial distortion model, once the fascial band is completely untwisted, the symptoms are eliminated because the distortion no longer exists. FDM techniques therefore, are more than just another treatment option — they are potentially a cure.

The example of the pulled muscle involves a single presentation of only one of the six principal distortion types. However, it illustrates how different interpretations of anatomical injuries lead to different treatment choices and dramatically different treatment results. But before exploring each of the fascial distortion types, there are several fascial concepts that should be addressed.

THE UBIQUITOUS FASCIA

Fascia is found throughout the body and constitutes a tremendous amount of sheer weight and bulk. As the primary connective tissue, it presents in many well-known forms such as tendons, ligaments, retinacula, fascial bands, aponeuroses, adhesions, pericardial sac, pleura, meninges, and the perimysium and epimysium of muscles, as well as many other

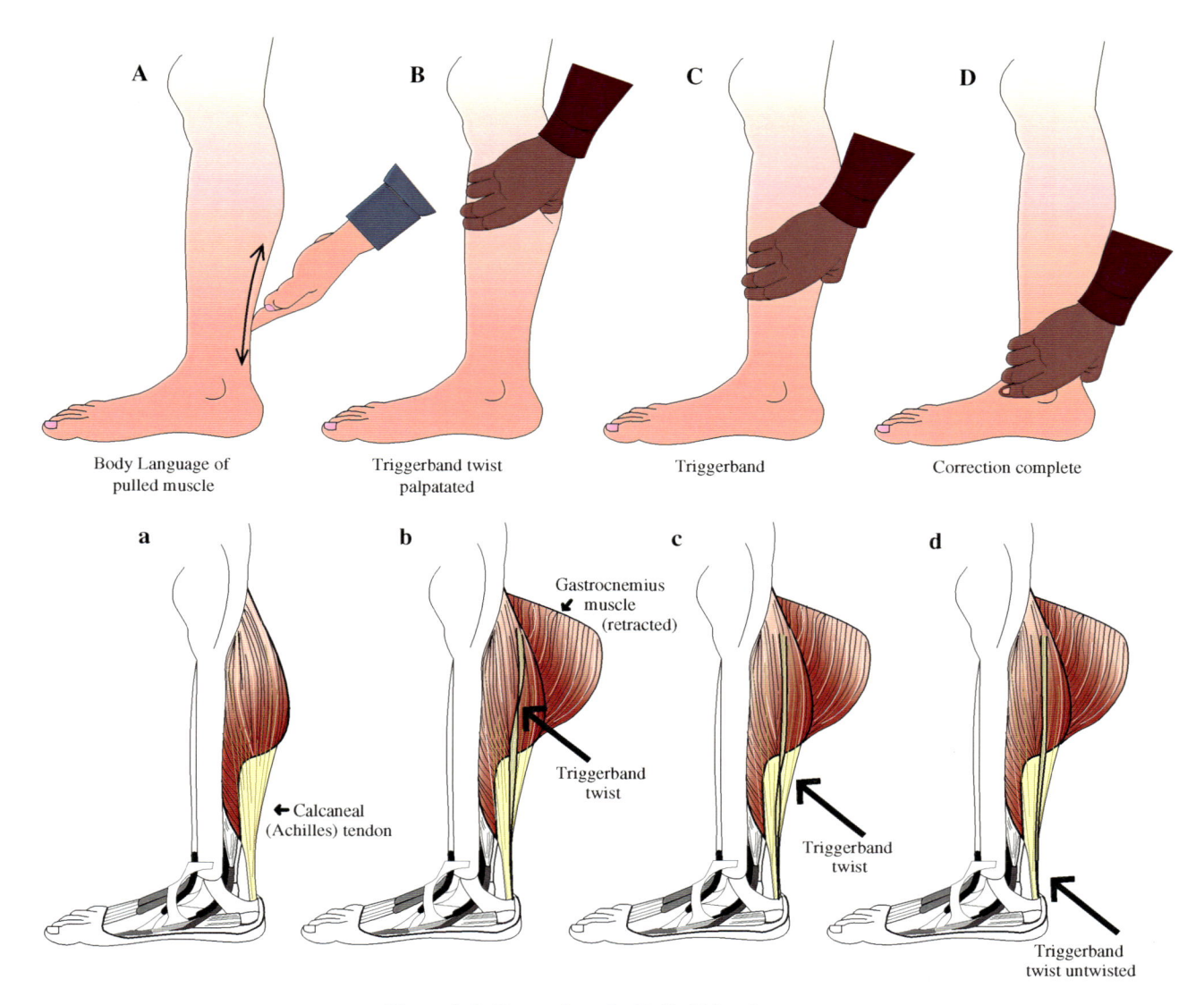

Figure 1-2. Correction of a Pulled Muscle

In the FDM, parallel fascial fibers that transverse through a muscle can become twisted. These distorted bands (known as triggerbands) are responsible for the subjective symptoms and physical findings of what is commonly referred to as a *pulled muscle*. In the pulled calf muscle (shown above) a triggerband has formed deep in the gastrocnemius muscle.

- A. Patient demonstrates body language associated with a pulled muscle (sweeping motion with fingers along triggerband pathway)
- a. Twisted fibers of fascial band hidden deep within belly of gastrocnemius muscle

- B. Twisted fibers palpated – triggerband technique (smoothing out twisted fibers with treating thumb along entire fascial band pathway) initiated by physician
- b. Anatomical location of triggerband twist within belly of gastrocnemius muscle (superficial layers of muscle fictitiously retracted for visualization)

- C. Triggerband twist pulled out of muscle and onto calcaneal tendon (symptoms of pulled muscle resolved but symptoms of tendonitis created)
- c. Triggerband twist within fibers of calcaneal tendon

D/d. Correction complete – twisted fibers of fascial band/tendon are untwisted – patient is asymptomatic

structures. In addition to connecting, fascia surrounds, engulfs, encases, separates, compartmentalizes, divides, protects, insulates, and buffers bones, nerves, muscles, and other tissues. In fact, each individual muscle fiber is sheathed with fascia, as is each and every individual muscle bundle, and each and every muscle, as well as every group of muscles.

FASCIA: THE LIVING TISSUE

Fascial bands are made up of parallel fibers that transmit forces to neurological centers. In this way, fascia acts as a sensor of mechanical tension. An analogy of this is our own clothing which has a similar capability. If something (or someone) should tug on our pant cuff but not directly touch any part of our body, we would still have a fair appreciation of both the location and nature of the stimulus. This is because the tension on the pant cuff is transmitted up the pant leg to the waist where the stimulus is integrated into the neurological system. In this way, when a pant cuff is tugged, we know whether it is from one of our young children attempting to get our attention or from a rambunctious pet parrot doing the same (this is a true-life experience!).

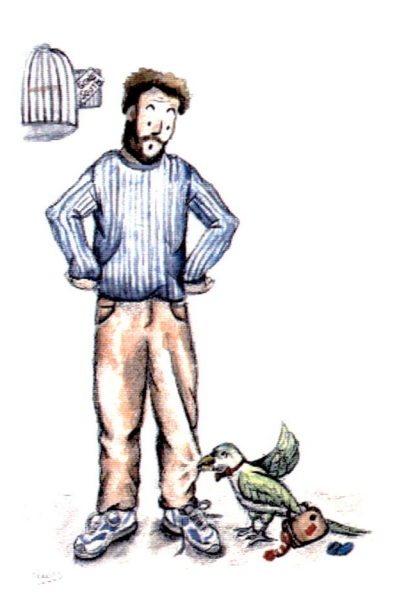

Figure 1-3. Clothing as a Mechanical Sensory System

Individual fibers of fascial bands (called *sub-bands*) maintain a natural tension. This tension force is called *pitch* and is unique for each particular fiber. When the sub-band is stimulated, it vibrates slightly. The greater the stimulus, the more it vibrates. The amount of resonance from each of the millions of sub-bands throughout the body supplies higher centers with in-depth and constant transmission of proprioceptive information.

In this way, fascial fibers function much as stringed musical instruments do. For example, a guitar or piano works on the principle of vibration. Each string has a specific length, and when stimulated, it vibrates at a precise frequency and causes a specific note to play.

Just as our ears hear music, our nervous system is interpreting fascial tension input. But, when the piano is out of tune, the expected frequency of the notes is changed. This is also the case with a distorted fascial band in which the *off-key* vibratory frequency is transmitted through the nervous system to the brain where it is deciphered as burning, tightness, pulling, or pain.

In addition to assisting in proprioception, fascial fibers are thought to have still other physiological functions. One of these is to coordinate motor movements and muscle contractions. The instantaneous changes in fascial fiber tension supply the nervous system with split-second information from every area of each small section of the muscle during contraction.

The connectedness of the fascial fibers can be thought of as a *continuity* of the tissue itself. For instance, although the lateral collateral ligament of the knee (LCL) and the iliotibial band (ITB) seem to be very different anatomical structures — they are in a sense one and the same. This is because some of the fibers of the LCL extend into the ITB and continue superiorly up to the iliac crest. The orthopathic consideration of continuity is that an injury to any of the connecting structures can have ramifications everywhere along the pathway.

In contrast to the continuity of fascial fibers, the FDM also considers the *continuum* of the structures. In this perception of anatomy, the fascia not only connects different tissue types, but the different tissues themselves are envisioned as compositional forms of each other. Bone and ligament, for instance, represent opposite ends of the continuum that is one anatomical structure. The concept of *anatomical continuum* is articulated in this book in Chapter 5. In the junction between ligament and bone, the fibers of the ligament merge into the osseous matrix and become the bone itself. This intermediate area (transition zone) has properties in between either adjacent tissue, and therefore is physically stiffer than ligament yet more flexible than bone.

The *physiological continuum* of fascia is demonstrated by the ligament/bone transition zone's ability to instantaneously shift its physical characteristics from bone-like to ligament-like, and vice versa, depending on the physical stresses encountered. This shifting of the continuum is analogous to the properties obtained when mixing cornstarch and water. In this amorphous substance a finger can be gently inserted and stirred (multidirectional forces are applied) and the mixture behaves as a liquid. But if a unidirectional force is introduced, such as from tapping, the mixture acts like a solid.

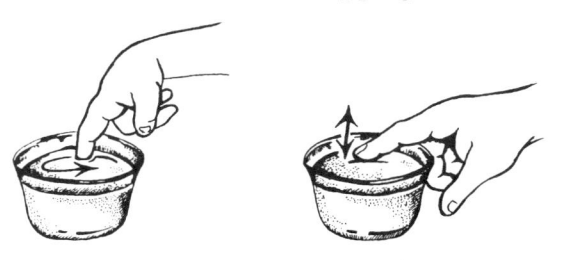

Figure 1-4. Cornstarch/Water Phenomenon

In the FDM, the fascial network, therefore, is not viewed as the hopelessly superfluous mesh of wasted complexity that so many suppose it to be. It is instead envisioned as a well-organized organ system in its own right. Besides the functions previously mentioned, the fascial system has the added duty of augmenting the circulatory and lymphatic systems in transporting bodily fluids. Through this *connective tissue highway*, bones and other tissues are constantly replenished with chemicals and nutrients. Thus fascial distortions not only physically restrict motion, alter proprioception, and inhibit muscle function, but also disrupt fascial fluid transport and thereby disturb the chemical balance of the associated tissues.

INFLAMMATION, FRACTURES, AND PAIN

Since fascia acts as a mechanical sensory system, it has within itself the capability of causing pain. However, restitution of the physically distorted fascia to its uninjured state anatomically eliminates that portion of pain production. A clinical example illustrates this point.

A 15 year old boy twisted his left ankle playing basketball two days before.
Chief Complaint: Ankle pain
Mechanism of Injury: "Heard it pop" when another player stepped on his foot. As he fell to the ground the leg twisted and the ankle buckled laterally.
Description of Discomfort:
1. Pulling tightness along lateral leg
2. Pain in spot on outside of ankle
3. Aching deep inside ankle (aggravated with full weight bearing)

Body Language exhibited when asked to "show where it hurts":
1. Sweeping motion with fingers along lateral distal leg
2. Points with one finger to spot of pain on lateral malleolus
3. Gently places hand over anterior ankle

Physical Findings:
- Walks tentatively with large ankle-to-knee brace and cannot completely bear weight without it
- Unable to place foot squarely on floor
- Bi-malleolar swelling
- Ecchymosis from ankle to toes
- Point tenderness of lateral malleolus
- Diminished dorsiflexion, eversion, and inversion

Radiological Findings:
- Non-displaced transverse fracture of mid-portion of lateral malleolus

Orthopedic Diagnosis: Ankle (distal fibula) fracture
Orthopathic Diagnosis: Ankle (distal fibula) fracture with:
1. Lateral ankle triggerband
2. Lateral ankle continuum distortion
3. Folding distortion of tibiofibular interosseous membrane

The standard orthopedic care for this injury involves casting or splinting, R.I.C.E., and anti-inflammatory and/or analgesic medicines. The purpose of the cast or splint is to keep the fractured segments from further separating, while R.I.C.E. and anti-inflammatory medicines are prescribed to reduce swelling. Crutches and splints are two additional options used to minimize the discomfort associated with ambulation.

However, this patient was treated orthopathically rather than orthopedically, meaning that manual manipulative treatments were done with the intent of correcting fascial distortions. Since a folding distortion of the interosseous membrane was presumed to be responsible for the pain deep in the joint and for keeping him from bearing full weight, it was treated first. This same distortion (see Figure 9-1 for visualization of interosseous membrane folding distortion of forearm) was also considered to be inhibiting the fractured segments from fully re-approximating. Two other distortions were then treated: the triggerband responsible for the pulling pain up the leg (see Figure 12-5), and the continuum distortion which caused the sharp pain near the fracture site (see Figure 5-2).

Once these distortions were corrected, the patient was immediately able to place his foot on the floor, bear full weight, stand on his toes, and walk at normal speed without a limp. No cast, splint, crutches, wrappings, or medicines were given. At subsequent rechecks or inquiries (two days, two weeks, and six weeks later) he continued to be walking well and remained pain-free.

Although this patient suffered a significant injury to his ankle, it was the distorted fascia that was responsible for his pain — not the fracture or inflammation. Furthermore, the orthopathic treatment he received accelerated the reunification of the lateral malleolus with its fractured segment by eliminating fascial distortions which were physically inhibiting re-approximation. And since the fascial structures were no longer impeding joint movement and muscle contractions, the ankle exhibited normal range of motion. Additionally, the treatment facilitated the re-absorption of interstitial swelling by restoring the fascial fluid transport system.

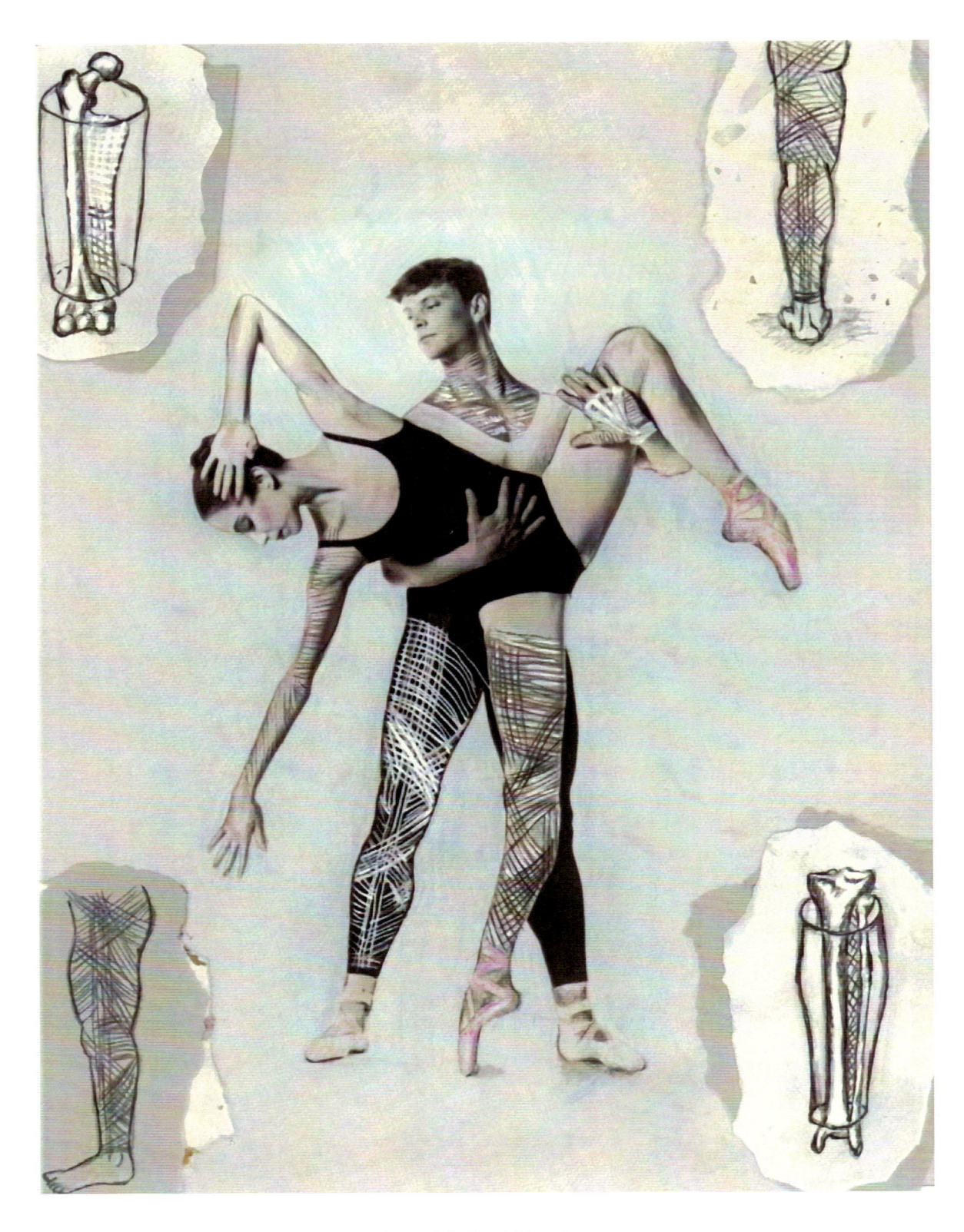

Figure 2-1. Fascial Bands

Maria Terezia Balogh and Todd Edson model some of the millions of fascial fibers found throughout the body. Injured fascial bands, which are called triggerbands, typically cause a burning or pulling pain that is inconsistent with previously described neurological, muscular, or dermatomal patterns. Drawing based on illustrations from Gerlach, U.J., and Lierse, W.: Functional Construction of the Superficial and Deep Fascia of the Lower Limb in Man. *Acta Anact* (Basel) 1990;139 (1):11-25.

Chapter 2

PRINCIPAL TYPES OF FASCIAL DISTORTIONS

In the fascial distortion model there are currently six principal types of fascial distortions:

Triggerband	—	distorted fascial band
Herniated Triggerpoint	—	abnormal protrusion of tissue through fascial plane
Continuum Distortion	—	alteration of transition zone between ligament, tendon, or other fascia and bone
Folding Distortion	—	three-dimensional alteration of fascial plane
Cylinder Distortion	—	overlapping of cylindric coils of superficial fascia
Tectonic Fixation	—	alteration in the ability of fascial surfaces to glide

---

Virtually every musculoskeletal injury from a pulled muscle to a frozen shoulder can be considered to be comprised of one or more of the above fascial distortions. The treatment strategy in the orthopathic approach is to determine which types of distortions are present in any given injury and to correct them. For instance in a sprained ankle, if the underlying injury is a continuum distortion, then we treat with continuum technique. If it is a triggerband sprained ankle, then triggerband technique should be utilized. And finally, if it is a folding sprained ankle, then only folding technique is expected to result in a desirable outcome.

This same philosophy is used over and over again on every musculoskeletal injury:
- Determine the fascial distortion types present
- Select and apply the corresponding fascial distortion techniques

Every principal fascial distortion type has certain characteristics that allow us to identify and appreciate it for what it is. Collectively these clinical traits give each of the principal types a unique *personality* with which we can become familiar. Discussed in this book are terms such as *burning*, *moving*, and *jumping* that are all key words patients use to convey information about their injuries.

TRIGGERBANDS: The most common of all, these are twisted or wrinkled fascial fibers that cause a *burning* or *pulling* pain along the course of the fascial band. Patients often subconsciously make a sweeping motion with their fingers along the involved pathway when describing their discomfort. (You can think of TB's as a twisted ribbon, a twisted shoulder harness, or a *Ziploc®* bag that has become unzipped.)
TREATMENT: Untwist the twisted fibers and iron out the wrinkle
NOTE: During treatment the pain can be moved along the course of the fascial band

HERNIATED TRIGGERPOINTS: Rarely found in the extremities, HTP's feel like "spongy marbles," and are almond-sized or smaller fascial herniations.
TREATMENT: Push the protruding tissue below the fascial plane

CONTINUUM DISTORTIONS: Think of these distortions as tiny injuries of the bone-ligament transition zone. Patients point to CD's with the tip of their finger and complain of pain in one spot.
TREATMENT: Force the osseous components in the transition zone to shift back into the bone

FOLDING DISTORTIONS: These injuries are similar to what happens to a road map that unfolds and then refolds in a contorted condition. Folding distortions hurt deep in the joint.
TREATMENT: Unfolding injuries – traction joint to allow the folding fascia to unfold and then refold less contorted
Refolding injuries – compress joint to overfold folding fascia which then springs back (unfolds) less contorted

CYLINDER DISTORTIONS: Anatomically reminiscent of a tangled *Slinky®* toy, cylinder distortions cause deep pain in a non-jointed area which cannot be reproduced or magnified with palpation.
TREATMENT: Untangle the overlapped coils of this superficial fascia
NOTE: Watch for the pathological phenomena of the pain *jumping* from one location to another

TECTONIC FIXATIONS: When patients complain that their joint is stiff or feels like it is a *quart low on oil*, they are describing a tectonic fixation. TF's are fascial surfaces which have lost their ability to glide.
TREATMENT:
1. Brute force is used to slide the fixated surfaces
2. Manipulative techniques are used to pump synovial fluid through the joint

Since fascia is present throughout the body, fascial distortions can occur virtually everywhere. For the purpose of this book, a sampling of injuries is listed below with the distortions most commonly present shown in the likelihood of their occurrence.

Sore Shoulders: Triggerbands
                                  Herniated triggerpoints
                                  Cylinder distortions
                                  Continuum distortions
                                  Folding distortions
                                  Tectonic fixations

Tennis Elbow: Triggerbands
                                  Continuum distortions

Long-Standing Elbow Pain:	Tectonic fixations Folding distortions Triggerbands
Carpal Tunnel Syndrome:	Cylinder distortions Triggerbands
Finger Sprains:	Folding distortions Triggerbands Continuum distortions Cylinder distortions
Neck Pain:	Triggerbands Tectonic fixations Herniated triggerpoints Folding distortions Continuum distortions
Upper Back Pain:	Tectonic fixations Triggerbands Cylinder distortions Folding distortions
Rib Fractures:	Continuum distortions Triggerbands
Fibromyalgia:	Triggerbands Cylinder distortions Folding distortions
Acute Low Back Pain:	Triggerbands Continuum distortions Folding distortions Tectonic fixations Cylinder distortions Herniated Triggerpoints
Long-Standing Low Back Pain:	Triggerbands Tectonic fixations Folding distortions
Long-Standing Hip Pain:	Tectonic fixations Folding distortions

Renal Colic Pain:	Herniated triggerpoints Triggerbands
Non-Organic Abdominal Pain:	Herniated triggerpoints Triggerbands
Biliary Colic:	Herniated triggerpoints Triggerbands
Groin Pulls:	Triggerbands
Knee Sprains:	Triggerbands Continuum distortions Folding distortions
Shin Splints:	Triggerbands Continuum distortions
Ankle Sprains:	Continuum distortions Triggerbands Folding distortions Cylinder distortions (if a splint is used)
Foot Sprains:	Cylinder distortions Folding distortions Continuum distortions Triggerbands (Note that in foot sprains all of the above are about equally common)

WHY USE FASCIAL DISTORTION TECHNIQUES?

In orthopathic medicine the treatment is selected according to the anatomical distortion present in the injury. Deciding which fascial distortion technique to use in any given injury then becomes obvious. For instance, if a triggerband is the underlying cause of an injury, then triggerband technique is chosen. In contrast, if the injury is the result of a continuum distortion, then continuum technique would be selected. And the same matching of distortion with technique applies to herniated triggerpoints, tectonic fixations, and folding and cylinder distortions. Although there are many other osteopathic and non-osteopathic therapies that are commonly used in the treatment of musculoskeletal injuries, only fascial distortion techniques are specifically designed to correct fascial distortions.

Chapter 3

Triggerbands and Triggerband Technique

Triggerbands are anatomical injuries to banded fascial tissues in which the fibers have become distorted (i.e., twisted, separated, torn, or wrinkled). The associated verbal description of burning or pulling pain along a linear course accompanied by the corresponding body language (sweeping motion with the fingers along the triggerband pathway), directs the corrective treatment specifically to the distorted fibers of the afflicted fascial band, ligament, or tendon.

Triggerband technique is the manual method for correcting distorted fascial bands. The goal of the treatment is to physically break fascial adhesions (if the injury is chronic), untwist the distorted band or sub-bands (individual fibers of the band), and re-approximate the torn fibers. In essence, triggerband technique is accomplished by *ironing out* the wrinkled fascia with the physician's thumb. And although there are several subtypes (see table in Addendum) all triggerbands are treated the same way, and that is with triggerband technique.

Triggerband Technique and the Zip Lock Analogy

When a physician encounters a patient in the office with a triggerband, he or she wants to know two things: what a triggerband feels like and exactly how to do triggerband technique. If the triggerband can't be identified and corrected, then the treatment will fail. As with all of the fascial distortion treatments, triggerband technique puts the skills of the physician *out on the line* where neither a treatment success nor a failure is easily hidden.

Perhaps the best way to describe what a triggerband feels like is to compare it to a Ziploc® plastic bag. Triggerbands feel and behave in a very similar manner. The zip lock portion of the bag is banded (like fascial bands) and the plastic fibers run along the length of the banded portion (again like fascial bands). When the bag is zipped tight, the fibers are all straight, in line, and approximated (same as fascial bands). But when the zip lock fibers are forcefully pulled apart, the fibers separate, the edges twist, and the ends of the Ziploc® bag are pulled closer together (just as with a triggerband). As the injurious force continues, the fibers separate farther, become more twisted, and the opening enlarges. If the force persists, the zip lock will become fully unzipped (for a triggerband *fully unzipped* means that the entire triggerband pathway is affected).

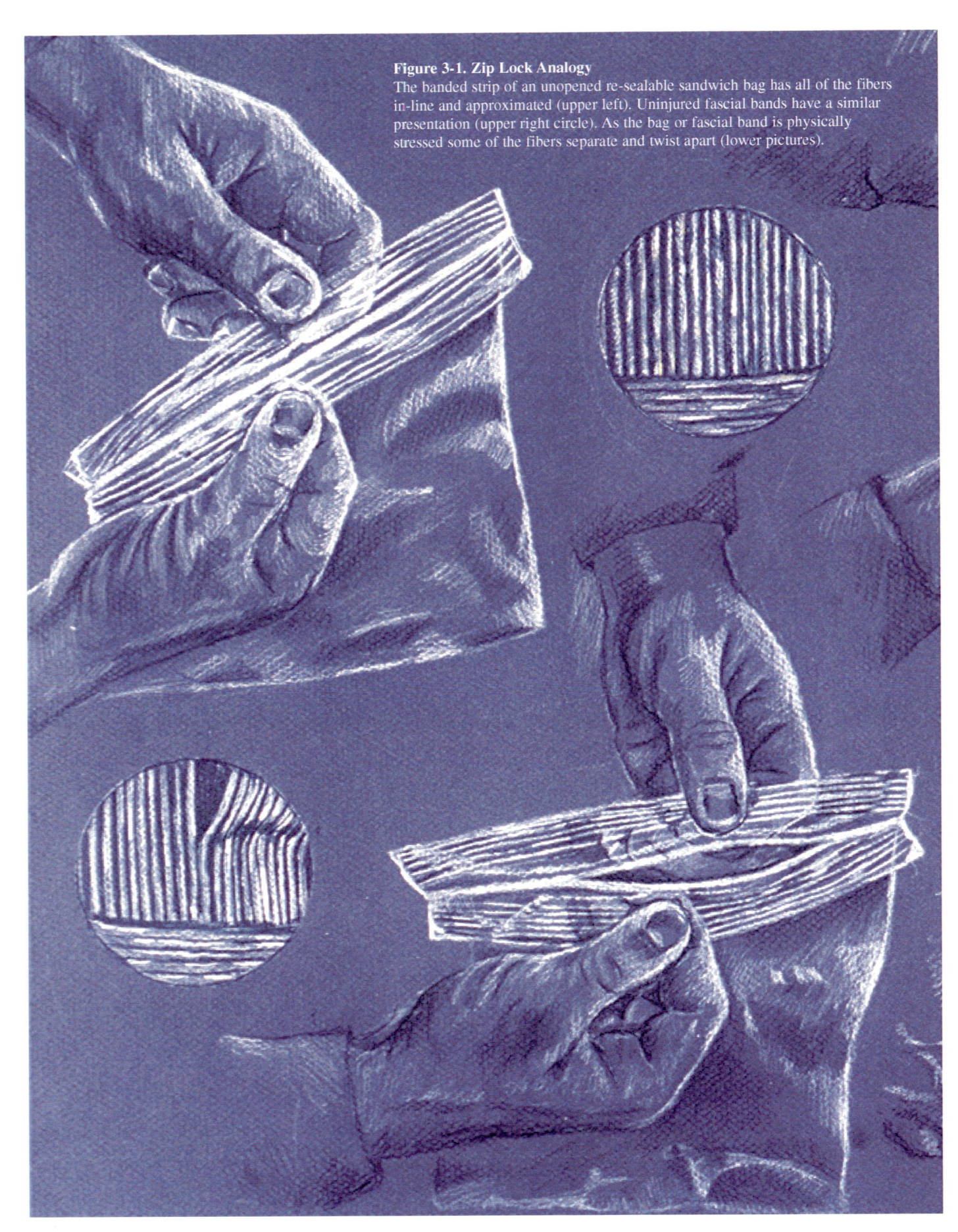

Figure 3-1. Zip Lock Analogy
The banded strip of an unopened re-sealable sandwich bag has all of the fibers in-line and approximated (upper left). Uninjured fascial bands have a similar presentation (upper right circle). As the bag or fascial band is physically stressed some of the fibers separate and twist apart (lower pictures).

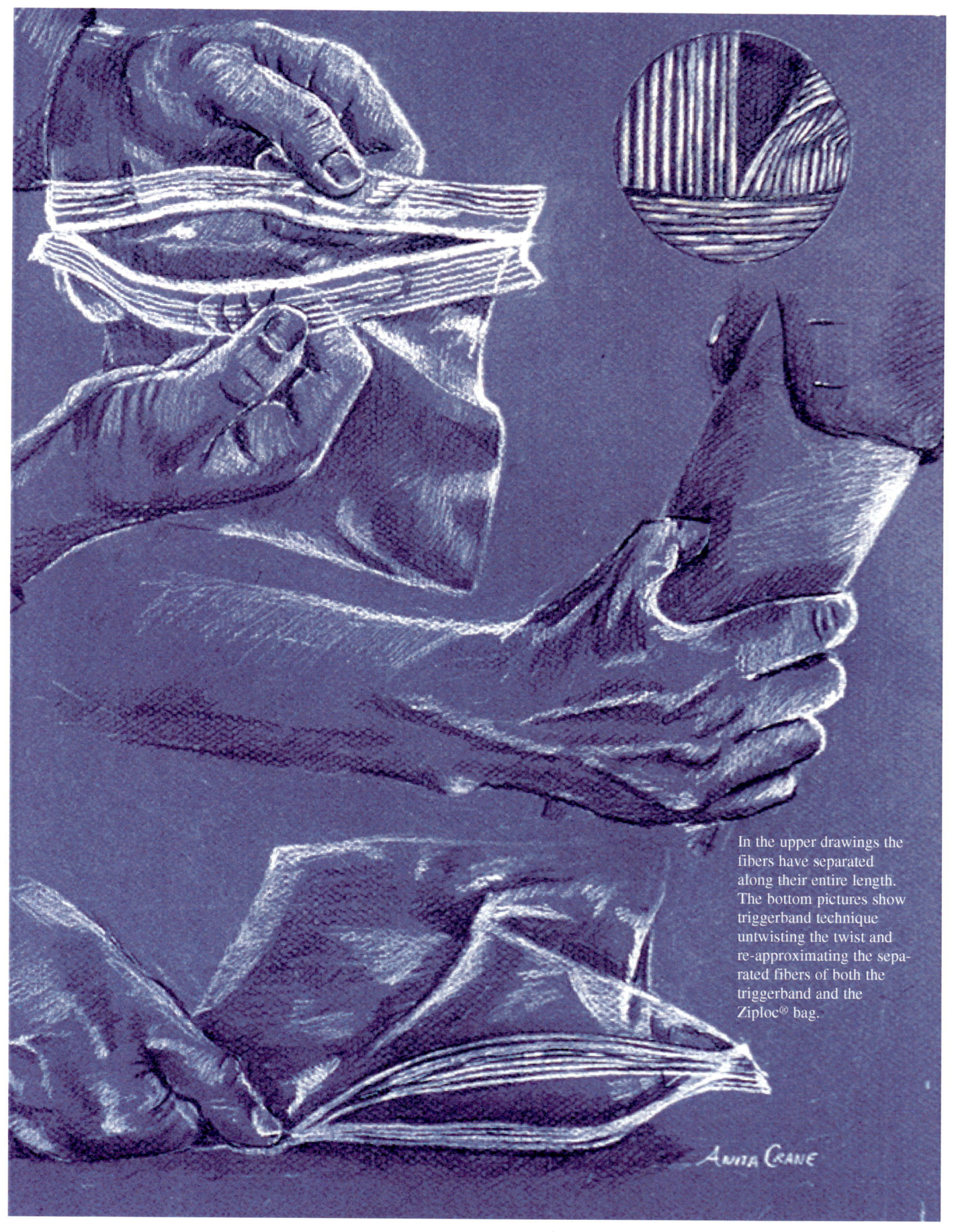

In the upper drawings the fibers have separated along their entire length. The bottom pictures show triggerband technique untwisting the twist and re-approximating the separated fibers of both the triggerband and the Ziploc® bag.

Anita Crane

Fascial bands behave exactly the same way as Ziploc® bags. They have banded fibers that are closely approximated and feel very much like the banded portion of the bag. When a force is encountered, the entire band may twist and torque slightly (just as with the Ziploc® bag). But if a shearing force accompanies the twisting motion, some fibers may be pulled apart from each other. If the force persists, then the separation between the fibers spreads throughout the entire length of the band.

RE-ZIPPING THE ZIPLOC® BAG

In this zip lock analogy of a triggerband, a distorted fascial band looks, feels, and behaves like an open or opening Ziploc® sandwich bag. In correcting a triggerband the thumb is used to re-approximate the separated fibers in the same manner as you would re-zip a Ziploc® bag.

To get the best feel for how a triggerband can be corrected, the reader should actually grab a Ziploc® bag from the kitchen drawer and lay it down on the table. With the bag unzipped and the ends secured in place with two heavy weights, you are ready to attempt to correct a *zip lock triggerband*. With the tip of your thumb (and with your eyes closed) feel for the distorted fibers. Then push the fibers back together along the entire length of the zip lock.

WHY TRIGGERBANDS STAY FIXED

Two questions frequently asked about triggerband technique are:
- "Why don't the fibers just separate again as soon as you push them back together?"
- "What's holding them in place?"

These questions apply equally well to the Ziploc® bag. But you can appreciate from your own experimenting that once re-zipped the seal is tight and only a force similar to the initial injury could cause the same separation.

When a triggerband is corrected it is *cured*. There is no need for healing time because once the fibers are re-approximated, they seal instantaneously. And just as the zip lock fibers can be pulled apart and sealed over and over again, with no appreciable loss of function, the same is also true with fascial bands.

TRIGGERBANDS AND CROSSLINKS

Fascial bands have one significant structural advantage over zip lock bags — crosslinks. Crosslinks hold the fibers of the band together in the same manner that chains bundle logs into a load for transportation on a truck. However, if sufficient external force is directed into the band, the crosslinks will fracture and the fascial fibers will separate.

Healing of the distorted fascial band occurs when the separated fibers are re-approximated and the ends of the fractured crosslinks reattach. The healing time for re-linking is almost immediate when the fascial fibers are in close proximity, but is extended if the fibers are not properly realigned.

If the injured fascial band is allowed to heal on its own, the fractured crosslinks reach out and re-link their broken segments, which then physically pull the separated fibers together and untwist the distorted fascial band. However, the danger in reattachment is that the wrong crosslinks may be united. If this occurs the fascial band is inappropriately anchored to a neighboring band which further decreases the flexibility of both structures. In the FDM, this mal-attached crosslink unit is called an *adhesion*. And from a clinical perspective, any injury which contains adhesions is considered to be *chronic*.

Acute triggerbands (i.e., those triggerband injuries without adhesions) have four possible futures:

1. Heal quickly (almost immediately) with triggerband technique
2. Heal slowly on their own (the crosslinks properly reattach by reaching out to their appropriate counterparts)
3. Not heal at all (the injury persists but because of physical exercise, the crosslinks don't reattach)
4. Become chronic (crosslinks attach to inappropriate structures)

Acute Triggerband   **ChronicTriggerband**

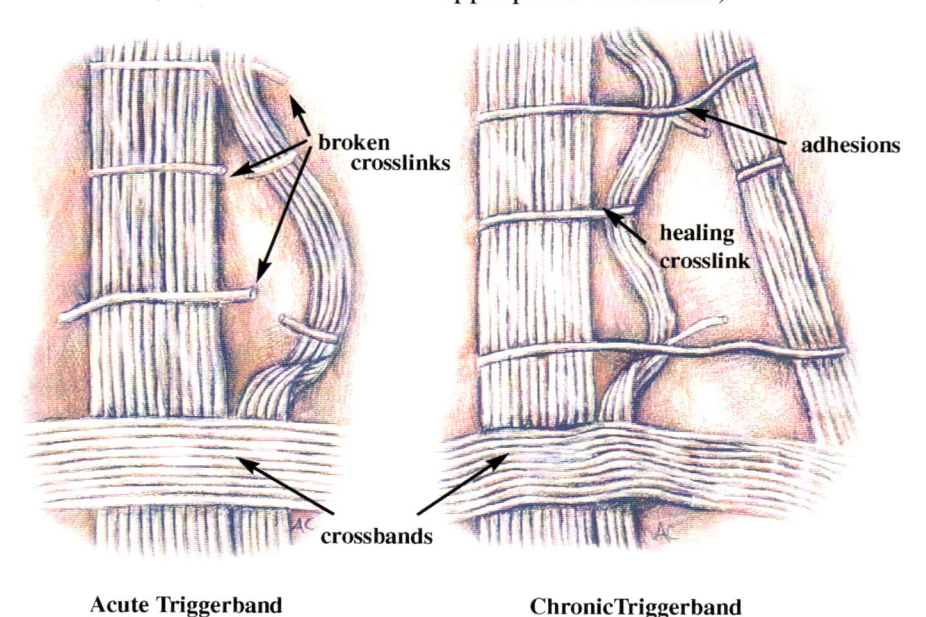

Figure 3-2. Acute and Chronic Triggerbands

In an acute triggerband (left) crosslinks have been fractured and some of the sub-bands (individual fibers) have twisted apart. Note that crossbands stop the fibers from tearing indefinitely and are the starting point for triggerband technique. If the torn crosslinks heal by attaching to structures other than their appropriate counterparts (right) they are called fascial *adhesions* and the injury is considered to be *chronic*.

CROSSBANDS

During an injury, fascial fibers can't tear indefinitely — what stops them are *crossbands*. These are anatomical structures present in the same plane that intersect the affected fascial band at an angle. Crossbands may be retinacula, fascial bands, other banded fascial structures, and even bone, any of which can stop the progression of separating fibers. Since the crossband fibers are at an angle to the triggerband, the sub-bands (individual fascial fibers of the fascial band) are more or less perpendicular to the vector of force. Generally speaking, only a traumatic global force as from an auto accident, or a specific force such as from a knife, could be expected to tear through the crossband at such an angle.

BODY LANGUAGE

The associated body language of patients with triggerbands is always the same: sweeping motion with the fingers along the triggerband pathway. Clinically, for instance, if someone complains of shoulder pain and makes a sweeping motion with the fingers along the bicipital groove (see Figure 11-1) we can be confident of not only the diagnosis of triggerband sore shoulder but that the involved triggerband is the anterior shoulder pathway.

In addition to determining the specific identity of a triggerband, the body language also is helpful in ascertaining the following:
- Direction of triggerband (affected fibers run parallel to the sweeping motion of the hand)
- Extent of pathway involved (the more sweeping the hand motion is, the farther along the pathway the fibers have separated)
- The deeper the triggerband is anatomically – the more firmly the person pushes into the fascia with his/her fingers

TREATING THE TRIGGERBAND PATHWAY

Triggerband technique includes the following steps:
1. Determining pathway
2. Palpating starting point
3. Re-zipping

DETERMINING THE PATHWAY

Since different people tend to have the same anatomical arrangement of fascial bands, triggerbands occur in consistent patterns called pathways. In the anterior shoulder pathway for example, the triggerband course is always the same — starting point on proximal anterior forearm and pathway that runs superiorly through the bicipital groove, up the lateral neck, and terminates at the mastoid on the same side.

Palpating the Starting Point

The starting point (SP) is the clinical beginning place from which triggerband technique is initiated. This tender anatomical roughening in the contour of the fascia occurs at the intersection of the afflicted fascial band with its corresponding crossband. In the anterior shoulder pathway, the starting point is located on the ventral forearm where the superiorly directed fibers junction with the horizontally oriented fibers of the bicipital aponeurosis.

To palpate the SP of the anterior shoulder pathway, the volar aspect of the treating thumb is laid across the forearm (pointing toward the antecubital fossa). And with increasing force the thumb prods the fascial tissue for the characteristic irregularity in tissue texture.

Re-Zipping the Triggerband

Once the starting point is localized, the interphalangeal thumb joint is flexed to a 90° angle so that the tuft of the distal phalanx is abutted against but just inferior to the starting point. Next, the thumb is held stationary while the fingers are rotated superiorly and grasp the elbow. As the thumb maintains steady and firm force it is dragged superiorly across the skin which irons out the fascial band. Note that the thumb rotates either medially or laterally during the process and it is helped superiorly by the pull of the rotating hand which is anchored by the fingers around the elbow.

Once the thumb reaches the antecubital fossa the hand creeps superiorly so that the fingers grasp the distal humerus and are pointing upward. The thumb is again dragged superiorly until the hand creeps up yet again. In this manner the thumb advances up the arm much like a car is hoisted with a jack. The treatment of the anterior shoulder pathway continues up the arm and through the bicipital groove, over the clavicle, up the lateral neck, and finally to the mastoid on the same side where the fibers terminate.

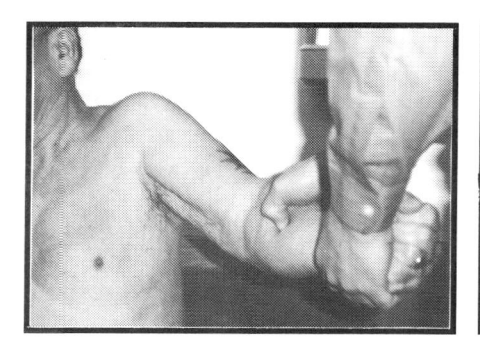

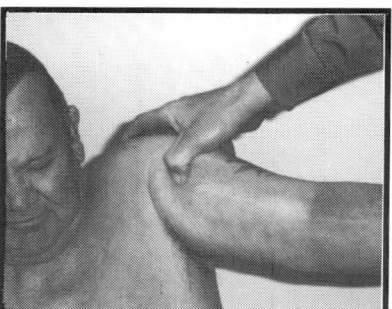

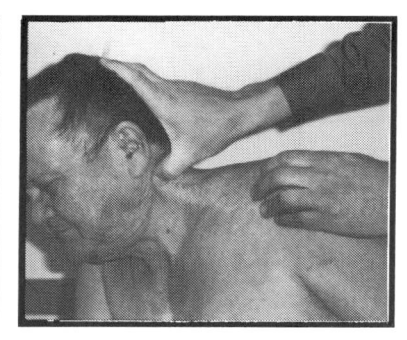

Figure 3-3. Triggerband Technique of the Anterior Shoulder Pathway

When using triggerband technique, it is important to stay on the pathway. If you are concerned that you have wandered off-course, ask the patient, "Am I still on it?" Even patients that have no idea of what you are talking about will be able to easily answer, "Yes, definitely," or "No, you lost it." If a patient says, "You left it," that means that you are no longer on the pathway.

TREATING THE CHRONIC TRIGGERBAND

Unlike acute triggerbands, chronic triggerbands don't zip right back together. They can't because adhesions are holding them in the unzipped position. They therefore require multiple treatments and more force to correct. And since adhesions are fractured, bruising and soreness from the initial treatments are expected. An additional approach in fracturing adhesions of chronic pain is the *comb*. This technique (also used for chronic pain of cylinder distortions) involves literally raking the skin with a steel comb. *Old Scratchy*, as it is affectionately called, fractures the small adhesions of fibromyalgia and is a valuable tool in the treatment of chronic pain.

NOT STARTING AT THE STARTING POINT

In treating the anterior shoulder pathway (or any pathway), it is generally best to begin at the starting point. This assures that the entire pathway is properly treated and that all of the lengthwise portion of the fibers has been re-approximated. However, in some patients it may not be necessary to treat the entire length of the pathway. Just as with the Ziploc® bag, the band may have only separated along a middle portion of its course. Starting in the middle requires greater palpatory skill but has the advantage of being a faster treatment. However, for those learning triggerband technique, it is suggested the entire pathway be treated every time until the technique is mastered.

TRIGGERBAND MOVEMENT

As stated earlier, triggerbands exhibit *movement*. This is best appreciated when a triggerband twist is moved up or down the course of the pathway during triggerband technique (see glossary term *Twisted Shoulder Harness Analogy*). In the triggerband sore shoulder, the bicipital groove may initially be sore, but that soreness can, with triggerband technique, be moved anywhere along the course of the triggerband pathway. The movement of pain is, of course, pathognomonic of a triggerband but has another ramification, namely that with triggerband technique it is possible to have *left the twist behind* when performing the technique. When this occurs, the patient has a new pain in an area he/she didn't have before. This is another reason for treating the whole triggerband pathway rather than only part of it.

MIXING TECHNIQUES AND CONCEPTS

When using triggerband technique, lotions, gels, or creams should not be applied. These reduce the friction on the skin which is needed to correct the underlying structures. Also it is important to appreciate triggerband technique as being a distinct treatment entity. It is not a form of massage, myofascial release, rolfing, acupressure, or any other modality. *Mixing* triggerband technique (or other FDM) concepts and practices with other techniques and concepts decreases its focus and thus its effectiveness.

Chapter 4

HERNIATED TRIGGERPOINTS AND HERNIATED TRIGGERPOINT THERAPY

Herniated triggerpoints (HTP's) are fascial distortions in which underlying tissue has protruded through an adjacent fascial plane and has become entrapped. These injuries are responsible for a wide range of painful complaints such as neck aches, sore shoulders, renal colic pain, abdominal pain, buttock strain, and behind-the-eye headaches. The three most commonly encountered HTP's are: *supraclavicular*, *bull's-eye*, and *abdominal*.

The anatomical goal of herniated triggerpoint therapy is to force the entrapped tissue below the fascial plane with pressure from the physician's thumb. The three components of therapy include:
1. Palpating the distortion
2. Applying pressure
3. Milking the release

SCHTP

Since the supraclavicular herniated triggerpoint is so prevalent it can be thought of as the *type specimen* for the group. The SCHTP is an almond-sized protrusion of tissue found in the indented space between the clavicle and the superior margin of the scapula. It is the usual culprit of thoracic tightness between the shoulder and neck, one-sided headaches where the head is tilted to the side of pain, and in approximately one half the cases of acute sore shoulders in which abduction is completely or partially lost.

The body language for the SCHTP is always the same — fingers pushing directly into the supraclavicular fossa (see Figure 11-1). The clinical findings closely match the symptoms:
- If the patient complains of upper back tightness, then the palpatory expectation is of tightened thoracic fascia
- If the complaint is instead a headache or neck ache, then we can expect slow or diminished neck rotation
- If the complaint is shoulder pain, there is likely to be diminished shoulder abduction or internal rotation (see Chapter 11)

To palpate the supraclavicular herniated triggerpoint the thumb-tip presses into the fossa until it encounters an irregularity in the tissues which may feel like a spongy marble. But be aware that no two are exactly alike! In fact some protrusions occur in the middle portion of the fossa and are relatively soft, while others are more medially located (even abutted up against C7 or T1) and firmer (almost almond-like in hardness).

In treating the SCHTP the patient is laid supine (sitting and prone are alternate positions) with the physician seated at the head-end of the table. The corresponding thumb, i.e., right thumb treats right SCHTP (secondary approach is left thumb for right SCHTP), applies pressure into the supraclavicular fossa and feels for the protruding tissue. Once palpated, firm pressure is directed into the most tender portion of the distortion as force from the volar aspect of the distal phalanx is increased. The thumb pressure should be continuous and progressive. If necessary recruit the non-treating hand to help push!

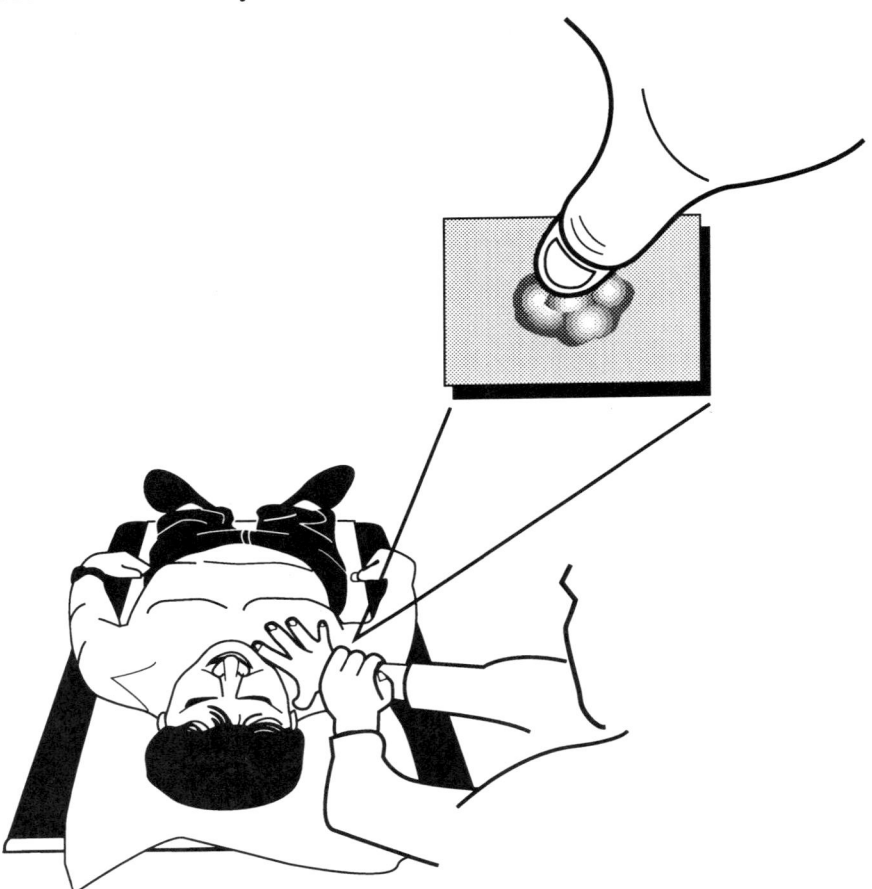

Figure 4-1. Herniated Triggerpoint Therapy of the SCHTP

The shortest part of the treatment is the release (5-10 seconds). It is defined as the *sensation experienced by physician and patient as the protruding tissue is physically drawn below the fascial plane*. To the treating doctor the release palpates as first a softening in consistency and then a lessening in size of the HTP. To the patient the release feels like a melting. The final process of herniated triggerpoint therapy is called *milking*. It is designed to coax even the smallest portions of the herniated tissue below the fascial plane by rocking the thumb back and forth during the release. Note that when first learning herniated triggerpoint therapy it may take the osteopath as long as 30 seconds to two minutes to complete the treatment. Most of this time is spent on locating the HTP and applying pressure.

One colorful way to envision herniated triggerpoint therapy is to think of the *cows through the barn door analogy*. In this metaphor, cows are coming home from pasture and need to be herded through a narrow door into the barn. Three ways to maximize efficiency are:
1. Line up all the cows in a row head-to-tail – this keeps them from crowding together and blocking the entrance
2. Physically shove each cow through the door instead of allowing them to meander into the barn at their own pace
3. Widen the door

In herniated triggerpoint therapy the protruding tissue is analogous to the cows. So to maximize treatment:
1. Use the thumb to line up the irregular protruding tissue so that one part at a time can be pushed through the fascial plane (one cow walks through at a time)
2. Use sufficient force – don't wait for the tissue to be pulled through on its own (kick the cows through the doorway!)
3. Have a second person traction the same-sided arm at a 30° angle to the body (see Figure 11-5) to increase the size of the fossa (make the barn door wider)

Figure 4-2. Cows Through the Barn Door Analogy

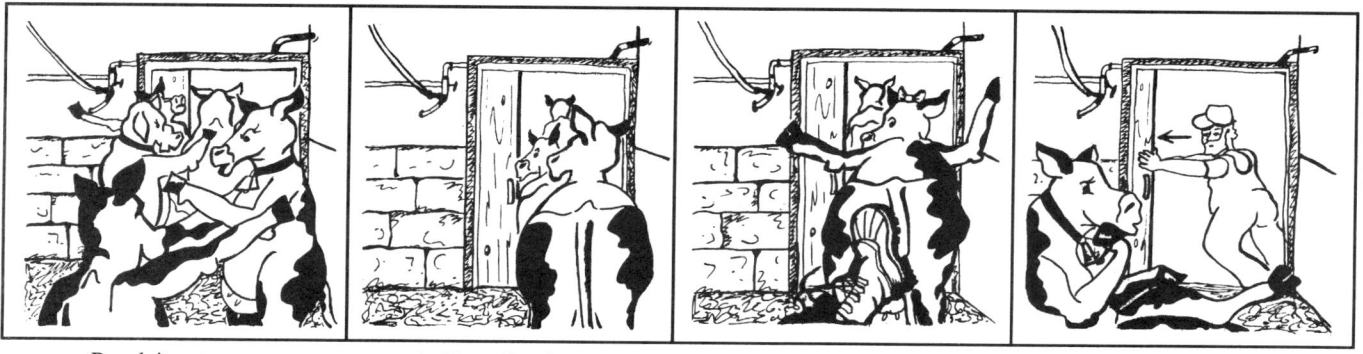

Recalcitrant cows outside barn　　1. Cows lined up　　2. Cows shoved into barn　　3. Barn door opened fully

BULL'S-EYE HTP

The bull's-eye herniated triggerpoint is found in the middle or lateral gluteal area and is a frequent cause of not only hip and gluteal pain, but also what many patients describe as "low back pain." Treatment consists of herniated triggerpoint therapy standing (with the patient leaning against a counter top), seated in a chair (with the affected buttock over the side of the seat), or prone. Note that the bull's-eye HTP is deep within the gluteal tissue so don't be concerned about pushing too hard. The goal of herniated triggerpoint therapy of the bull's-eye is the same as it is for the SCHTP — force protruding tissue below the fascial plane. The thumb-tip is again directed into the distortion until the protrusion is felt (the patient will know even if you don't!) and force is applied and held until the release.

ABDOMINAL HTP'S

Abdominal herniated triggerpoint therapy (along with triggerband technique) is a clinical and practical adjunct procedure for relieving or diminishing the biting pain and aching discomfort associated with pancreatitis, biliary colic, pelvic pain, and appendicitis. Although it is *not a substitute for medical evaluation or surgical treatment*, it anatomically corrects a portion of the pain-producing elements of an acute abdomen and therefore offers the physician (and patient) an effective non-pharmaceutical pain-killing supplement to narcotic analgesics.

Abdominal HTP's are located deep within the abdominal cavity and are easily appreciated by the patient upon palpation (they hurt!). Associated areas of discomfort include:
- Pancreatitis – left upper quadrant and epigastric areas
- Biliary colic – right upper quadrant
- Pelvic pain – pelvis
- Appendicitis – McBurney's point

Treatment consists of herniated triggerpoint therapy, i.e., pushing the thumb deep into the abdomen to first locate and then correct the herniated triggerpoint. However the anatomical backdrop in the abdomen complicates the treatment because there is nothing firm behind the HTP to push against. To give the thumb a background resistance, the direction of force can be altered slightly to bring the HTP against a firmer anatomical surface (such as a muscle). This is done by lifting or moving the entire plane of fascia with the opposite hand and then redirecting the force from the treating thumb into the resistance. The HTP is held until release which should result in a significant and immediate reduction in pain. After the first HTP is eliminated the patient is reevaluated:

1. No change in pain – the correction was not made, or the orthopathic impression was wrong (re-treat or reconsider diagnosis)
2. Reduction in pain – other uncorrected HTP's or triggerbands are concurrently present (treat remaining distortions; continue medical/surgical evaluation and treatment)
3. Complete relief of pain – orthopathic treatment was successful (continue medical/surgical evaluation and treatment)

It should be noted that aortic aneurysms, bleeding disorders, ruptured viscus, and a variety of other conditions are absolute contraindications to herniated triggerpoint therapy (or triggerband technique) in the abdomen.

Chapter 5

CONTINUUM DISTORTIONS AND CONTINUUM TECHNIQUE

When the transition zone between ligament, tendon, or other fascial structure, and bone loses its ability to structurally respond to external forces, this is called a continuum distortion. The presenting body language of this third principal fascial distortion type is distinct and obvious — pointing with one finger to the spot(s) of pain. And although some chronic injuries contain continuum distortions, the bulk of these exquisitely tender disruptions of the ligament/bone junction are found in acute injuries. Ankle sprains, cervical strains, sore shoulders, and sacroiliac pain are but a few examples of continuum injuries encountered daily in the emergency room setting.

The treatment of continuum distortions is with pressure from the thumb-tip directed into the transition zone. The correction is made when the osseous components are forced to *shift* back into the bone. And although this approach initially seems straightforward, the technical success of the treatment is dependent upon an appreciation of continuum theory.

CONTINUUM THEORY

Since, in the fascial distortion model, ligament and bone are envisioned as two opposite ends of one anatomical spectrum, both structures are seen as merely compositional forms of each other. Bone is therefore a fascial tissue with a large percentage of osseous material, while ligament is a fascial tissue with minimal bony products. And in the junction between them where the fibers of ligament blend into bone, there is an area which has both osseous and ligamentous physical properties. This intermediate section is called the *transition zone*.

In its neutral state this transition zone (TZ) has physical properties in between ligament and bone, i.e., it is more flexible than bone but more rigid than ligament. However, within the continuum theory the TZ is considered to have an additional physiological capability of instantly responding to external forces by altering the percentage of its osseous components. This shifting of bony components in and out of the transition zone gives the ligament/bone unit the capacity to make precise and computer-like structural responses to potentially injurious forces and thereby diminish the incidence of fractures and ligamental tears.

In the course of our daily lives, at any given moment the external forces that the ligament/bone junction encounter determine the percentage of osseous components that inhabit the transition zone. For instance, when the ligament and bone are subjected to unidirectional forces (such as from compression), osseous components are pulled from the bone into the TZ. However, if the ligament/bone junction instead encounters multidirectional forces (such as from circumducting a joint), osseous components shift back into the bone. The osseous configuration is therefore stronger (but stiffer), which protects the ligamental insertion from buckling, whereas the less strong but more flexible ligamental configuration shields against ligamental tears. It is this shifting of the continuum back and forth through the transition zone which gives our bones and ligaments the facility to minimize serious injuries.

Continuum distortions occur when a portion of the transition zone is subjected to a unidirectional force at the same time as another portion of the same zone encounters a multidirectional force. The result is that the transition zone splits its identity — one part becomes osseous and the other ligamental. These dual forces hold the TZ in two dichotomous states which, if one of the forces is extreme enough, may cause the responding section of the zone to *overshift* — meaning that so much osseous material is pushed in one direction, that even after the forces cease, that portion of the zone is unable to transfer sufficient bony components to be able to shift back into the neutral state. This imbalance in the transition zone between bone and ligament disrupts function of the ligament (some fibers are stiff, while others are flexible), and transmits to the brain uneven mechanical sensory information which is interpreted as pain.

Thus, continuum distortions can be thought of as a breakdown in the adaptive ability of the transition zone to shift. Therefore, when the injured transition zone encounters new forces that require the opposite configuration, that portion of the zone is incapable of responding (i.e., shifting). Since the TZ can become stuck in either the osseous or ligamental configuration, there are two subtypes of continuum distortions:

1. Everted (ECD) – Portion of transition zone is stuck in the osseous configuration, i.e., osseous components can't shift *from the transition zone into the bone*
2. Inverted (ICD) – Portion of transition zone is stuck in the ligamental configuration, i.e., osseous components can't shift *into the transition zone from the bone*

How To Do Continuum Technique

Continuum technique is the manual method for correcting continuum distortions. Note that the continuum distortion itself is palpated as a small (approximately the size of a lentil) roughening in the tissues which is impressively tender. The actual treatment consists of applying firm and continuous pressure directly into the continuum distortion and forcing the transition zone to shift i.e., bony products are forced out of the transition zone and into the bone. The volar aspect of the physician's thumb directs and focuses force into the altered transition zone which is held until the shifting occurs.

Figure 5-1. Continuum Distortions and the Ice/Slush/Water Analogy

In the FDM, ligament and bone are considered to be a continuum of one anatomical entity. In the ice/slush/water analogy the ligamental fibers (top of drawings) are the water, the transition zone between the ligament and bone is the slush, and the bone (bottom of drawings) is the ice. Far left diagram shows the transition zone in the neutral state.

When the ligament/bone unit encounters forces from several different directions, the transition zone shifts into the flexible ligamental configuration (middle left). But if the force is instead from one direction, the transition zone shifts into the stronger osseous configuration (middle right).

However, continuum distortions form when the transition zone is subjected to both singular and multidirectional forces. The uneven stresses result in one portion of the zone shifting into the ligamental configuration and the other being held in the osseous configuration. If one of the external forces is sufficient, the corresponding portion of the transition zone will overshift and become stuck in that configuration (far right drawing).

Two pathological possibilities exist:
1. Uninjured portion of transition zone (yellow) has shifted back into the ligamental configuration while the adjacent injured part (blue) is held in the osseous configuration (everted subtype)
2. Uninjured portion (blue) has shifted back into the osseous state while the injured part (yellow) is held in the ligamental state (inverted subtype)

Treatment of ECD's:

1. Apply pressure with thumb onto the *stuck* osseous portion of transition zone (blue) and physically force it to shift

Treatment of ICD's:*

1. Apply pressure with thumb onto the *unstuck* osseous portion of transition zone (blue) and physically force it to shift
2. Thrusting manipulation of the joint to draw osseous components into the ligamental fibers (yellow)

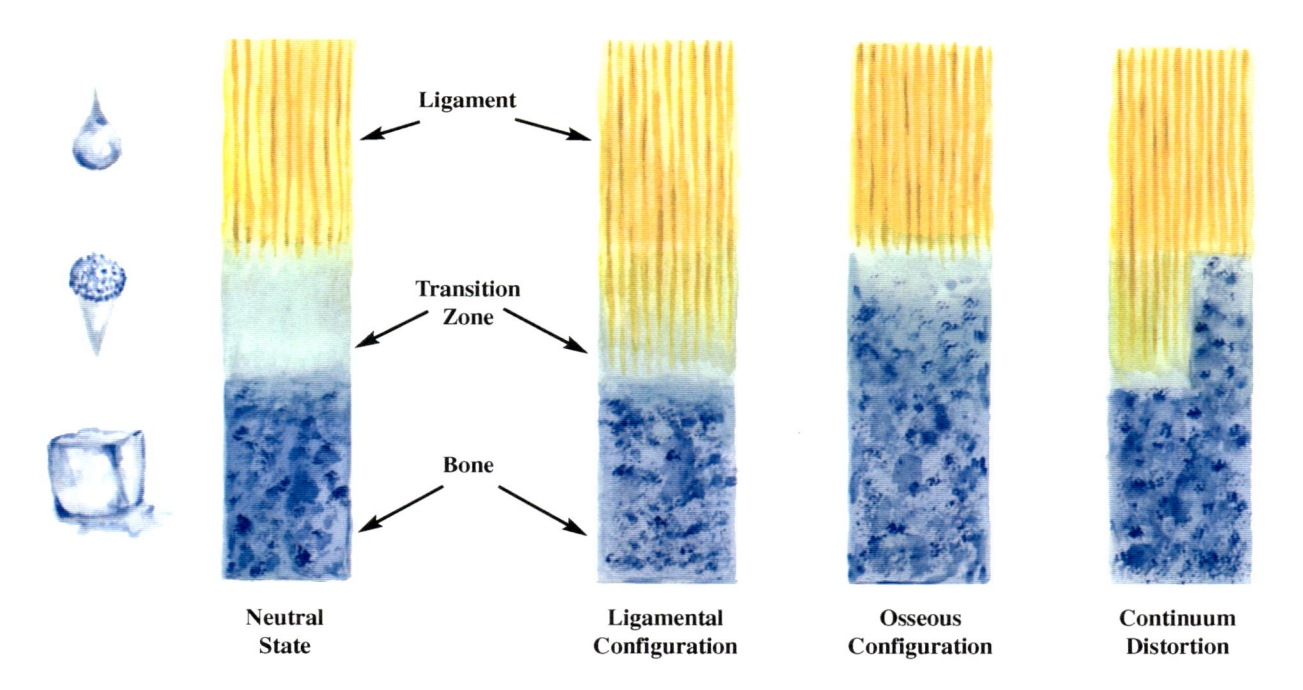

| Neutral State | Ligamental Configuration | Osseous Configuration | Continuum Distortion |

*Future treatments of ICD's will involve more precise methods of pulling or suctioning bony elements into the transition zone.

To find the continuum distortion, the tip of the thumb worms its way through the peripheral tissue until it rests on the distortion. Force is focused directly into the most painful spot. If the patient should say, "That's not too bad," this implies that the direction of force is off-mark. Readjust the thumb-tip and change the angle of force to maximize the pain and hold in that position until the transition zone shifts (normally this requires 5-30 seconds of holding firm pressure before the shifting occurs). The release itself lasts from 1-5 seconds and feels to both doctor and patient like a button slipping into a buttonhole. Note that once the zone shifts, the patient will immediately relate a dramatic reduction in discomfort.

The force used in continuum technique should be of opposite direction to the force that caused the injury, but of equal intensity. For instance, in a continuum sprained ankle, the calcaneofibular ligament typically exhibits a continuum distortion because bony components were pulled into it when the ankle buckled laterally. If the CD occurs at the origin of the ligament, the direction of force from the treating thumb should be directed into the attachment of the ligament on the calcaneus (see Figure 5-2). However, if the CD occurs at the insertion of the ligament, the direction of force from the treating thumb should be directed into the attachment of the ligament on the fibula. In either case, the amount of treatment force should be significant because the force of injury was significant.

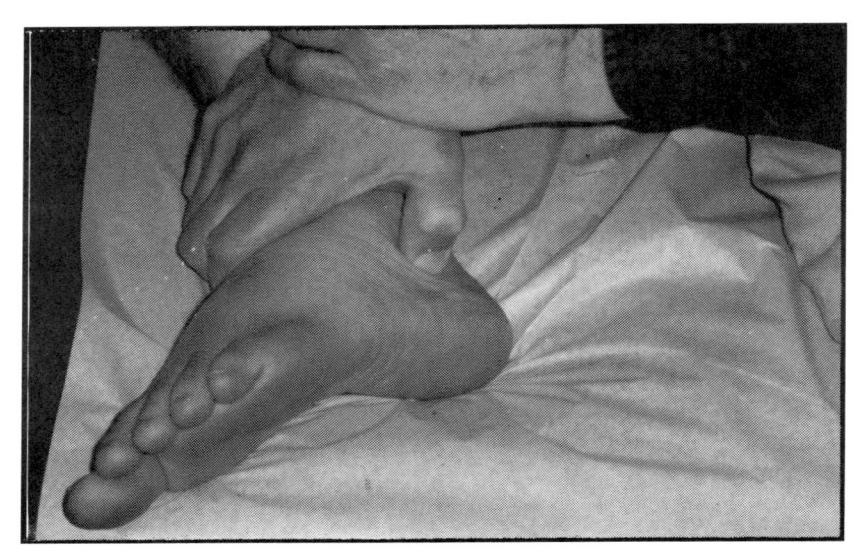

Figure 5-2. Treatment of Lateral Ankle Continuum Distortion

Once the continuum distortion has resolved, it no longer exists, and the injured area is immediately improved (i.e., there is dramatically less pain and the neighboring joint demonstrates increased strength with greater mobility). Note that the two most significant factors of a successful continuum treatment are:
1. Proper direction
2. Adequate force

THE ALL-OR-NONE PRINCIPLE

Continuum technique works on the *all-or-none* principle. Either the transition zone shifted, or it didn't. There is no in-between. If the direction or intensity of force is insufficient, then the transition zone won't shift. With continuum technique you cannot get a partial result because either the transition zone shifted, or it didn't.

EVERTED AND INVERTED CONTINUUM DISTORTIONS

Continuum technique is best suited to correct everted continuum distortions. These are the injuries in which excess osseous components have been pulled into, and are *stuck*, in a portion of the transition zone between ligament and bone. Although the remaining portions of the transition zone may shift back and forth freely as different forces are applied, the injured portion remains stuck in the everted configuration.

Since in inverted continuum distortions, the osseous components need to be pulled out of the bone, not pushed in, they typically respond less well to continuum technique. However, continuum technique may still correct them. This is because the uninjured area (i.e., the *unstuck*, more osseous portion of the transition zone) can be forced to shift into the ligamentous state. Because that portion is then in the same configuration as the stuck portion next to it, it may *pull* the stuck portion with it when it shifts again into the neutral state.

Although inverted continuum distortions initially respond well to continuum technique, a few hours or days later some seem to reoccur. This re-emergence of the signs and symptoms is possible because in an inverted treatment (unlike an everted correction) the unstuck portion of the transition zone has shifted, not the stuck part. So later, when the zone shifts again, it may do so as a whole unit (meaning that the treatment was successful), or only part of it may shift and the other part stays stuck (meaning that the treatment needs to be repeated).

Note that HVLA can be utilized as an adjunct treatment to continuum technique for the correction of inverted continuum distortions (particularly those of the sacroiliac joint, and cervical, thoracic, and lumbar spines). Reason – the manipulation tugs on the bony matrix and pulls osseous components into the transition zone. However, it should be made clear that HVLA is contraindicated in treating everted continuum distortions because:
1. It can make the distortion more symptomatic by pulling additional bony products into the already overshifted osseous portion of the transition zone
2. During the first 24 hours following correction of an ECD, the zone is not completely structurally united and HVLA may force osseous material into the previously corrected portion of the zone and thus recreate the ECD

WHAT TO DO AFTER CONTINUUM TECHNIQUE

Once a continuum distortion is corrected, there is little aftercare. If the patient is pain-free and the injured area has normal motion and strength, then there are no automatic restrictions. For an athlete with a sprained ankle, he or she may be allowed to continue participating immediately (or in a day or two, depending on the comfort level of the treating physician). For all continuum injuries ice massage is a *big yes* as an adjunct treatment since it seems to be helpful in reducing generalized discomfort. Heat in the first week and thrusting manipulation of everted distortions in the first 24 hours are two *big no's*.

CONTINUUM TREATMENT FAILURES

If the treatment result was less than dramatic, then either the technique was improperly applied, or additional types of fascial distortions (including continuum distortions) may be present. Remember that continuum technique works on an all-or-none principle. There are no partial results. If proper direction and force are held and the distortion won't release this is most likely because it is not a continuum distortion, but a small triggerband. To determine if it is a triggerband, push the distortion at a slight angle to see if it moves. If it does, then it is a triggerband and should be treated with triggerband technique.

Some injuries consist of many continuum distortions. If so, a successful treatment is just a question of numbers; the more that are corrected, the better the result. If necessary, bring the patient back the next day and *don't take any prisoners*.

Chapter 6

FOLDING DISTORTIONS AND FOLDING TECHNIQUE

When fascia around a joint becomes distorted from either traction or compression forces, this is called a folding distortion. These three-dimensional injuries of the fascial plane hurt deep within the joint and diminish the ability of the fascia to protect against pulling or pushing injuries. Within the FDM there are two subtypes of folding distortions — *unfolding* and *refolding*. Unfolding distortions occur when a pulling and twisting force is introduced into a joint and the fascia unfolds, torques, and refolds contorted. The main structural ramification of this injury is that the fascia can't refold completely. Refolding injuries, in contrast, occur when the fascia becomes jammed or compressed onto itself and then can't unfold completely.

FOLDING DISTORTION SUBTYPES

Unfolding and refolding distortions can be distinguished from each other by:

1. Mechanism of injury
2. Direction of force which reduces or exacerbates the pain (unfolding injuries feel better with traction and worse with compression, while refolding injuries feel better with compression and worse with traction)
3. Therapeutic response to folding techniques (unfoldings respond to unfolding techniques, i.e., traction and/or traction/thrust; whereas refoldings respond to refolding techniques, i.e., compression and/or compression/thrust)

Note that folding techniques of any kind should not be painful. If they are this means that the direction of thrusting force is wrong and needs to be reversed, i.e., changed from traction to compression or from compression to traction.

UNFOLDING DISTORTIONS

Unfolding distortions hurt deep within the joint and result from the limb or other body part being yanked. In the shoulder, the most common mechanism of injury is of a pet pulling on its harness or leash. The unknowing partners in these incidents are generally horses and dogs. In the case of the horse, the accident occurs as the equine suddenly throws its head forward and the force of pull is directed through the reins and into its owner's shoulder. In the case of the dog, the accident occurs as the canine lurches forward at an unexpected moment, jerking both its leash and its owner's shoulder (see Figure 6-1).

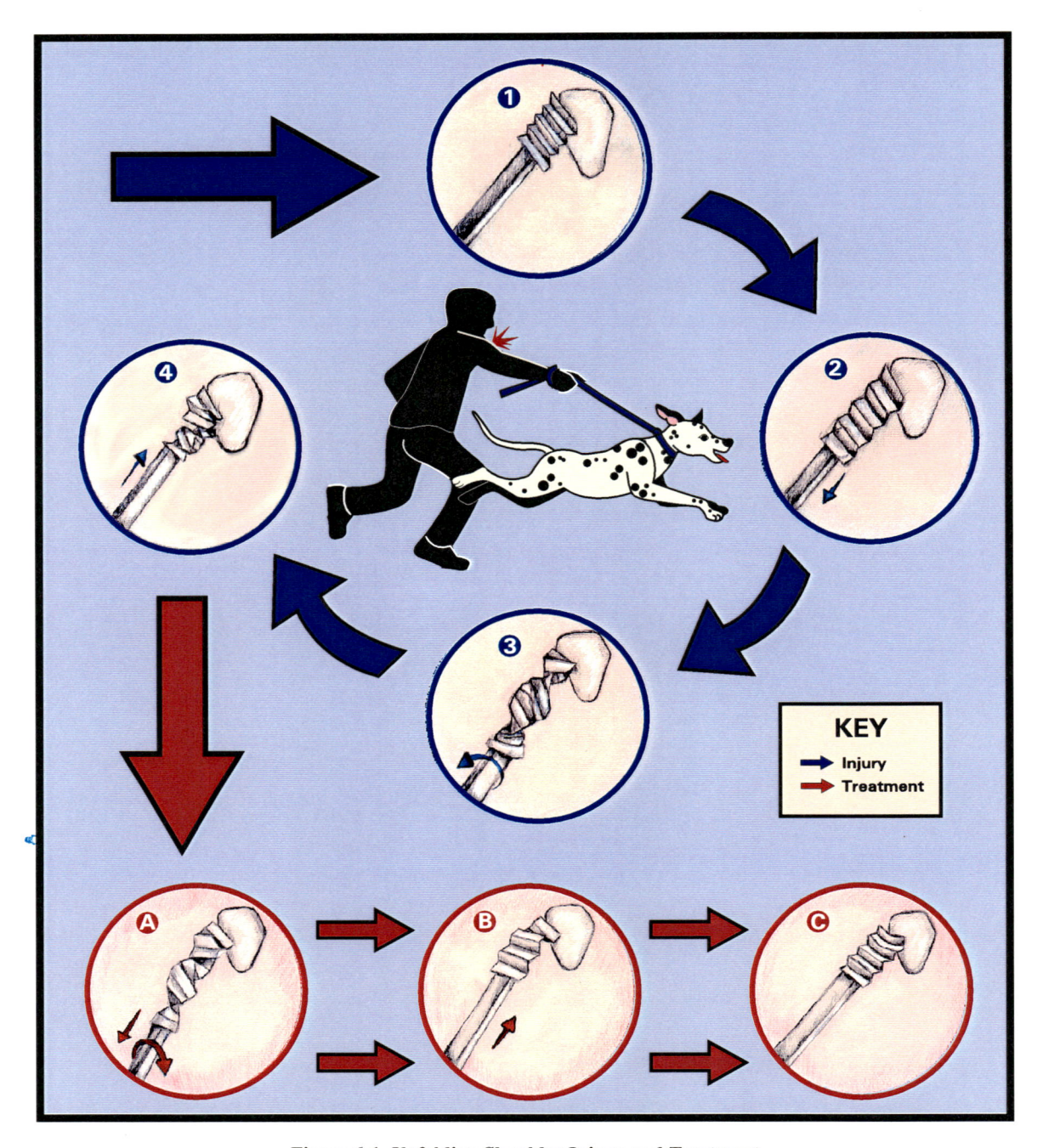

Figure 6-1. Unfolding Shoulder Injury and Treatment

Mechanism of Injury

1. Schematic of uninjured folding fascia
2. Fascia unfolds as shoulder is yanked
3. Flinching from pain causes the fascia to torque
4. The torqued fascia refolds contorted

Treatment of Unfolding Distortion

A. Treatment consists of reinitiating traction and untorquing the torqued folding fascia
B. Once the correction is made, traction is terminated and the fascia begins to refold
C. The corrected fascia, now refolded, is no longer contorted

The treatment of unfolding distortions is conceptually similar to that for reducing a dislocated shoulder, only less force is necessary for resolution. To treat, traction is applied to the affected limb until the fascia unfolds and then refolds into its proper configuration. With unfolding technique the injured limb is subjected to traction and torque in a variety of different directions. First, traction is applied in one direction and then another until the desired result is achieved. As traction is maintained, a slight twisting motion should be initiated to help untorque the contorted fascia. Unfolding technique is concluded when either the correction has been made or the doctor fatigues. Since this is a labor-intensive therapy, several sessions may be required to correct the distortion. A second approach to treating unfolding distortions is the whip technique, which is discussed in the chapter on tectonic fixations and tectonic technique.

When an unfolding correction is made, the tension on the joint diminishes. This lessening of tension may feel to the patient or doctor as a *release*. Some unfolding distortions, in contrast, resolve with a *clunk*. Others correct with a *staccato manipulation*, which is felt or heard as a series of rapid pops as the fascia unfolds and refolds. If the injury has become chronic (i.e., fascial adhesions have formed), then triggerband technique should precede unfolding technique.

Clinically, unfolding distortions are responsible for sore shoulders, sprained ankles, low back pain, and knee sprains. In addition, they are very typically present in the interosseous membrane following a wrist or ankle fracture (see Figure 9-1).

REFOLDING DISTORTIONS

Refolding distortions hurt deep in the joint (like unfoldings) and occur when the fascia around a joint becomes physically over-compressed. This *squashing* of the folding fascia compresses it so much that it is then unable to unfold completely. In the shoulder, the most common mechanism of a refolding injury is slipping on the ice and falling on an outstretched hand. Providing that the wrist or elbow isn't fractured, the force of the hand hitting the ground is transferred up the extremity to the folding fascia surrounding the gleno-humeral joint.

The treatment of refoldings is to approximate and untorque the mis-compressed fascia. Compression along with an accompanying thrust refolds the tissue still more tightly and allows it to spring back (i.e., unfold) less contorted once the force is terminated.

Note that unfolding corrections *pop* or *clunk* during the traction/thrust procedure, but with refolding corrections the audible *click* is generally not heard or felt until immediately after the compression/thrust. Since it is the snapping apart of the fascial planes that is responsible for the sound, refolding corrections aren't often audibly appreciated until a second or two after the thrust — which is the time it takes for the contorted fascia to first refold and then unfold.

Figure 6-2. Refolding Shoulder Injury and Treatment
Treat with compression/thrust of the humerus into the glenoid fossa

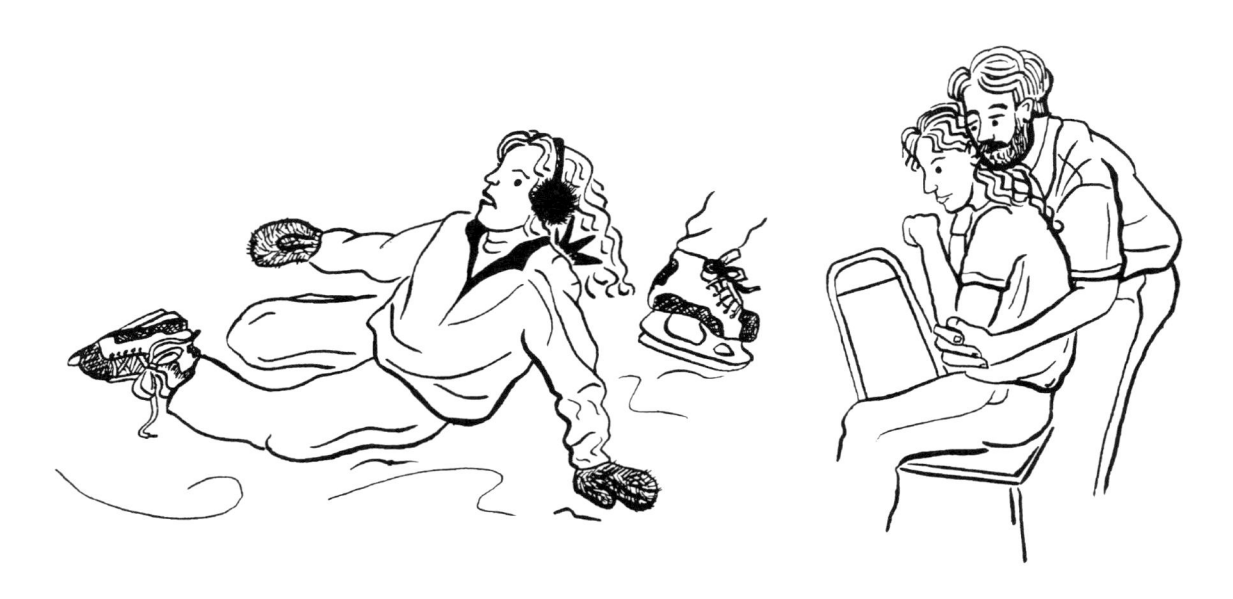

Clinical Examples of Unfolding and Refolding Injuries

Shoulder Pain
1. Horse bucked its head forward and jerked reins which owner was holding
   Dx: Unfolding injury
   PE: Pain reduced by traction, and increased by pushing head of humerus into glenoid fossa
   Tx: Unfolding technique, i.e., traction/thrust

2. Ice skater falls on outstretched arm
   Dx: Refolding injury
   PE: Pain reduced by pushing upper arm into shoulder, and increased by pulling on arm
   Tx: Refolding technique, i.e., compression/thrust of humerus into glenoid fossa

Knee Pain
3. Walked down steps in swimming pool and missed a step so that the knee hyperextended and then twisted
   Dx: Unfolding injury
   Hx: Pain increased by walking and relieved by resting
   Tx: Unfolding technique, i.e., traction/thrust

4. Walked down steps, anticipated a final step that wasn't there, and foot came down hard onto floor
   Dx: Refolding injury
   Hx: Most stiff after resting, stiffness decreases with walking
   Tx: Refolding technique, i.e., compression/thrust

Low Back Pain
5. Auto accident in which there was a head-on collision – airbag protected head and face, seatbelt restrained passenger in seat
   Dx: Unfolding injury
   PE: Discomfort is increased by compression and relieved by stretching
   Tx: Chair traction/thrust manipulation

6. Tripped down stairs and fell on buttocks
   Dx: Refolding injury
   PE: Stretching lumbar spine hurts, but pushing hard down on shoulders diminishes low back pain
   Tx: Chair compression/thrust manipulation
   Avoid stretching, traction, and hallelujah maneuver

UNFOLDING AND REFOLDING COMBINATION INJURIES

Joints may become injured from concurrent compression and traction forces that simultaneously unfold and twist one portion of the fascia and compress and overfold another portion. The currently preferred treatment approach of these combination folding distortions is to first refold the folding fascia and then unfold it. To augment this refolding/unfolding process, compress and then traction the joint repeatedly until the folding fascia manipulates (i.e., an articular snap or a series of snaps is heard or felt as the fascia first refolds and then quickly unfolds).

CERVICAL, THORACIC, AND LUMBAR FOLDING INJURIES

During a folding injury to the spine such as from an auto accident, the paravertebral fascia becomes either stretched upwards and refolds contorted, or compressed downwards and can't unfold properly. Symptoms of either subtype include diffuse pain and tightness throughout the involved spinal segments. Treatment for neck, as well as thoracic, and lumbar folding injuries consists of first correcting other distortions that are present (particularly triggerbands with adhesions if the injury is chronic) and then utilizing either traction/thrust for unfolding injuries or compression/thrust for refoldings. Note that inversion therapy (discussed shortly) is reserved for patients who do not respond to manual folding techniques.

Cervical Folding Manipulations

If a patient is to be treated for an acute folding neck injury in the supine position, the physician sits at the head-end of the table. If instead it is felt that the patient would be more comfortable sitting, the doctor stands behind or just to the side of the chair. In either case, the principles of treatment are similar.

In an unfolding correction, the actual treatment begins with the introduction of a firm superiorly directed traction force into the occiput. This pulling force is maintained for five seconds or so before a high-velocity thrusting manipulation is performed. The thrusting manipulation can be of two types:
1. Straight traction in which the physician's hands quickly tug the occiput in a superior direction
2. Rotation

The preferred hand arrangement for the rotational thrust is the same whether on the seated or supine patient — the thrusting thumb is placed on the fixated cervical transverse process and the index and middle finger are positioned along the angle of the jaw. If the left side of the neck is to be manipulated, the right hand continues to traction as the left hand rotates the neck to the right until the physiological barrier is engaged. Then a rapid thrusting force from the thumb is directed into the transverse process. The vector of force follows along the mandible. It should be remembered that this is an unfolding manipulation, so traction should be maintained throughout the procedure. Care must be taken to avoid pinching the ear.

In refolding cervical manipulations, the hand position with the patient seated is such that the non-thrusting hand pushes downward, as the thrusting hand delivers the rotational manipulation. In the supine position both hands compress the neck before and during the thrust. In either seated or supine refolding manipulations, it is advisable to compress for five seconds before the rotational manipulative forces are introduced.

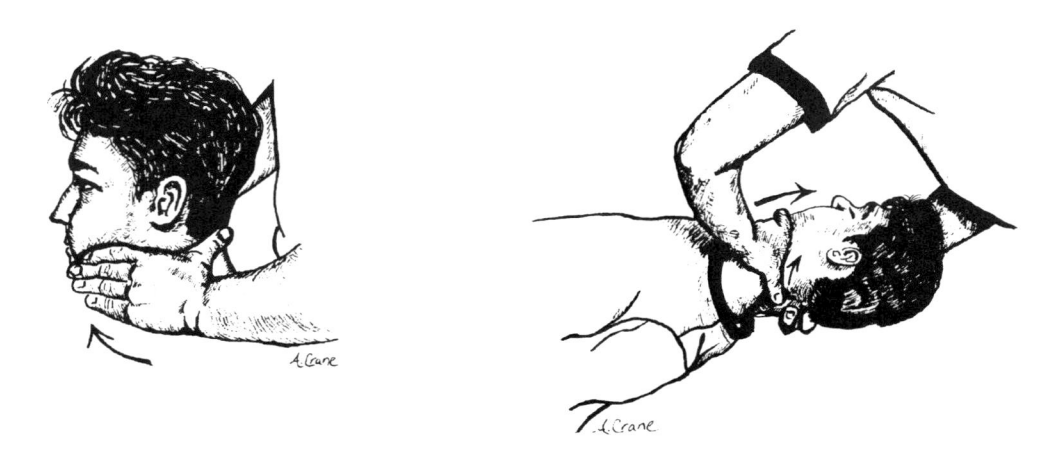

Figure 6-3. Folding/Thrusting Manipulations of the Cervical Spine

Thoracic Folding Manipulations

The most effective unfolding techniques for the thoracic spine are the hallelujah maneuver (upper thoracic) and the wall technique (lower thoracic). The most effective refolding technique for the thoracic spine (chair technique) is discussed in the section on lumbar folding manipulations. The hallelujah is performed with the patient standing or sitting and the shoulders externally rotated so that the elbows are pointing laterally. The doctor reaches from behind and places his/her hands through the triangular opening created by the patient's forearm, elbow, and neck. The treating fingers are then intertwined and placed on top of the patient's intertwined fingers. The thrusting maneuver is performed at the termination of a deep exhalation as the patient leans back into the physician. The finesse of this manipulation is such that the patient first falls limply backwards and then is smoothly but firmly lifted superiorly. Note that in Europe the hallelujah maneuver is better known as the *standing lift*.

The wall technique is performed with the patient standing, facing and leaning against a wall. The feet are brought to within several inches of the wall and the head rests on a pillow and is turned to either the right or left. A double pisiform hand position is taken so that the osteopath's left lateral hand and left pisiform traction the left paravertebral fascia, while the right lateral hand and pisiform traction the right paravertebral fascia. The hands, forearms, and even the doctor's chest can be used to traction and thrust the fascia. The direction of the thrust itself is toward the patient's chin. It should be emphasized that to be successful with this technique the direction of the traction and thrust should be as superiorly as possible. (The physician may wish to cushion his/her chest with a pillow or life preserver.)

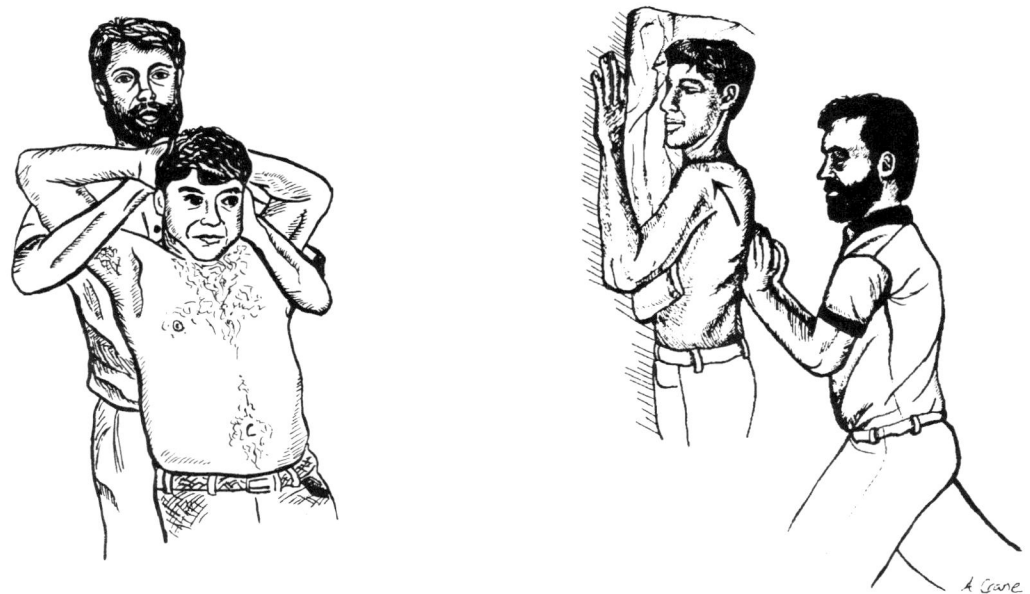

Figure 6-4. Hallelujah Maneuver (left) and Wall Technique (right)

Lumbar Folding Manipulations

Unfolding techniques: In general the treatment of lumbar unfolding strains currently involves either utilizing traction/thrust manipulations or inversion therapy. Traction/thrust involves high-velocity low-amplitude osteopathic manipulation (HVLA) coupled with traction. From a clinical perspective, less serious injuries respond best to traction/thrust, whereas extensive, diffuse, and long-standing injuries may require inversion therapy (see following section).

Although there are several thrusting manipulations which can be employed in the treatment of simple lumbar unfolding injuries, keep in mind the necessity of traction. One particularly effective method is commonly referred to as the chair technique. In this procedure, the patient sits backwards in a chair (i.e., straddles) so that he/she is facing towards the wall. The feet are tucked inside the legs of the chair that are closest to the wall and the forearms are crossed so that each hand can hold onto the opposite shoulder.

To make the correction, the osteopath stands behind the patient and reaches around with the non-thrusting hand and grips one or both of the elbows. The palm of the thrusting hand is placed over the transverse process and paravertebral fascia of the area to be manipulated. Simultaneously, both hands of the physician are used to traction and extend the spine. Once traction is maximized, the spine is rotated until the physiological barrier is reached. (When treating the right lumbar spine the physician's right hand is the thrusting hand.) Once the physiological barrier is engaged, a quick thrust is made by the palm of the treating hand. Please note that uncomplicated thoracic spine folding distortions can be corrected by a similar procedure.

Refolding techniques: The chair technique is also utilized to correct refolding distortions. The positioning is identical to that as described above and just as with an unfolding, the lumbar or thoracic spine can be manipulated. Note that with refolding corrections the thrust is preceded and accompanied by compression. The compression force is delivered through the hands, arms, shoulder (and at times even chin!) of the physician.

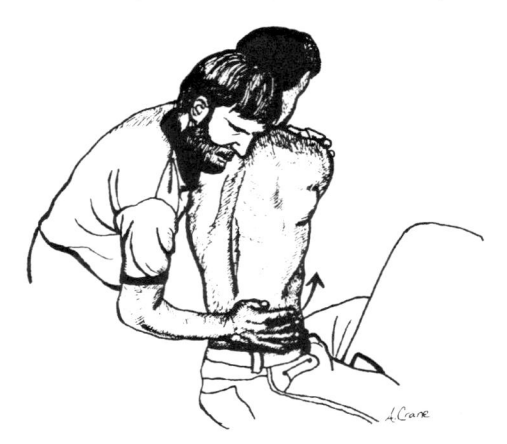

Figure 6-5. Chair Technique

INVERSION THERAPY

In extensive folding injuries of the thoracic and lumbar spine the sheer number of folding distortions renders folding/thrusting manipulations useless. Currently the preferred treatment of these stubborn injuries is to utilize the weight of the patient's body to force the paravertebral fascia to unfold or refold. These physician or physical therapist-guided, gravity-assisted folding techniques in which the patients are tilted or placed upside down (or close to it) are collectively known as inversion therapy.

With ball therapy the paravertebral fascia is unfolded by stretching the spine over a therapy ball. Multiple positions, such as flexion, extension, and side bending, engage different portions of the paravertebral fascia. If necessary, unfolding or refolding of the contorted fascia can be augmented by concurrent manual traction or compression of the spine or neck by the treating physician or physical therapist.

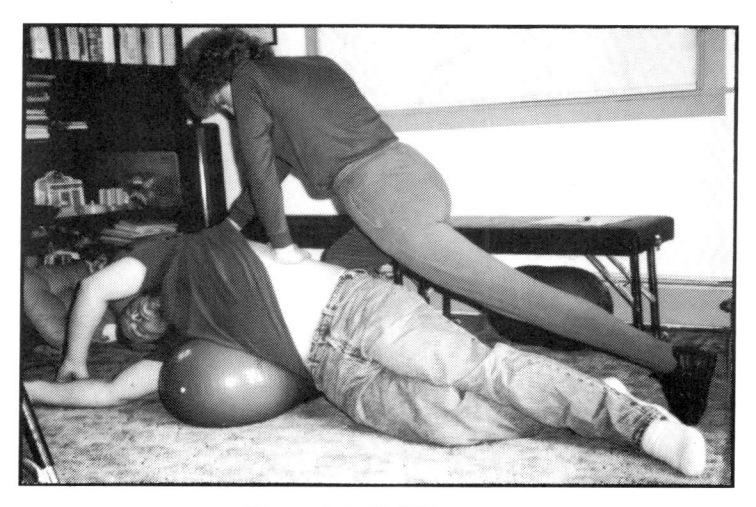

Figure 6-6. Ball Therapy

Inversion traction therapies are more generalized but aggressive forms of gravity-assisted folding techniques in which the patient is tipped to an upside-down or near upside-down position. If an inversion table is used (and there are no medical contraindications) the patient is placed supine onto the table and then slowly brought backwards to a 45-60° angle below the horizontal plane (see Figure 6-7, left photo).

Once the desired inverted position is achieved the patient is asked not to make any unnecessary movements of the spine or limbs for a minimum of fifteen seconds. This allows time for the paraspinal fascia to unfold in the neutral position. Following this short quiescent period the patient is encouraged to sidebend, rotate, and traction his or her own back to facilitate the unfolding of fascia that is contorted at an angle non-parallel to the spine. As with ball therapy, a concurrent traction or compression applied by the therapist or a thrusting manipulation by the osteopath may force additional unfolding or refolding.

Perhaps the most effective inversion therapy for the upper back and neck utilizes an apparatus in which the patient's hips and knees are flexed (see Figure 6-7, right photo). To direct the force of gravity into the thoracic and cervical spine, the patient is tipped forward until fully inverted. Just as with the other types of inversion treatments, the patient remains upside down for several minutes and can assist the procedure by pulling or pushing against the equipment. This varies the body posture and sequentially focuses gravitational and lateral forces throughout the affected paraspinal segments.

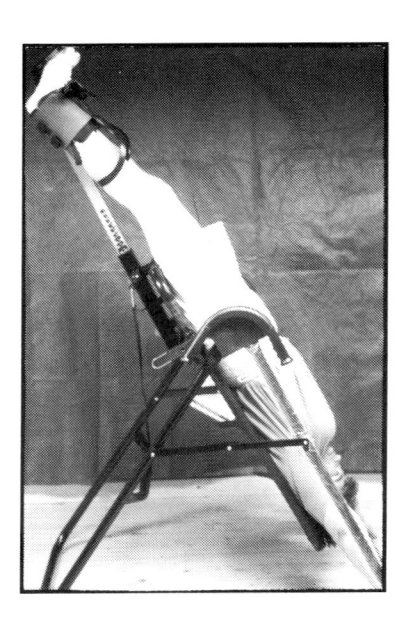

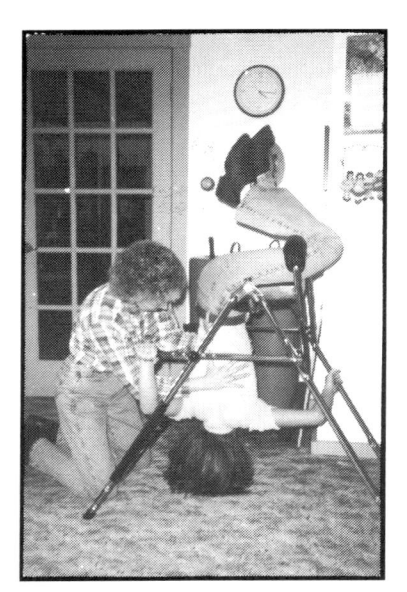

Figure 6-7. Inversion Traction

Please note that inversion therapy should only be performed under the direct supervision of a physician or physical therapist. Medical contraindications include hypertension, increased intracranial pressure, congestive heart failure, C.O.P.D., past history of cerebral hemorrhage, bleeding disorders, osteoporosis, glaucoma, vertigo, etc.

Warning: Positional changes should be made slowly to avoid the side effects of vertigo, nausea, and hypotension.

Chapter 7

CYLINDER DISTORTIONS AND CYLINDER TECHNIQUE

Anatomically, cylinder distortions are *tangled coils of circular fascia* which pathologically restrict motion by acting as a tourniquet around muscles. It is this entangling which inhibits the coils' ability to uncoil and recoil, thereby diminishing their resilience to absorb pulling and pushing forces.* Paradoxically, the deep pain in a non-jointed area which is so characteristic of cylinder distortions, involves cylindrically-oriented fascia which is surprisingly superficial.

Cylinder distortions are of particular interest to physicians because of their propensity to exhibit seemingly bizarre symptoms that mimic neurological conditions — such as tingling, numbness, and even reflex sympathetic dystrophy-like pain (see Case History #18). Also cylinder distortions in their most vicious forms present with symptoms that resemble orthopedic injuries — such as humeral head or neck fractures (see Chapter 11). But fortunately, most cylinder injuries are far less symptomatic and can be clinically recognized by the characteristic body language of *repetitively squeezing the affected soft tissues*.

The complaint of pain *jumping* from one area to another is expected with cylinder distortions, and indicates that the altered coils are being impeded in their rotation around the underlying muscles. Since the coils tangle in varying arrangements depending on the sequence of muscle contractions — the pain seems to periodically and abruptly change its anatomical location. In the FDM, this sudden geographical transposition of discomfort from one area to another is called the *jumping phenomenon*. Note that jumping:
- Is pathognomonic of cylinder distortions
- Occurs spontaneously on its own as the coils rotate with muscle contractions
- Can be induced with cylinder technique

Two mechanisms that distort circular fascia:
1. Twisting/traction forces separate coils which recoil tangled
2. Twisting/compression forces cause coils to overlap

From the above mechanisms the conditions we commonly refer to as carpal tunnel syndrome, tight muscles, upper arm strains, and low back spasms often occur.

---

*Note that folding fascia is the other fascial shock absorber. The difference between the two is that cylinder fascia protects muscles, whereas folding fascia defends against injurious forces to joints and bones.

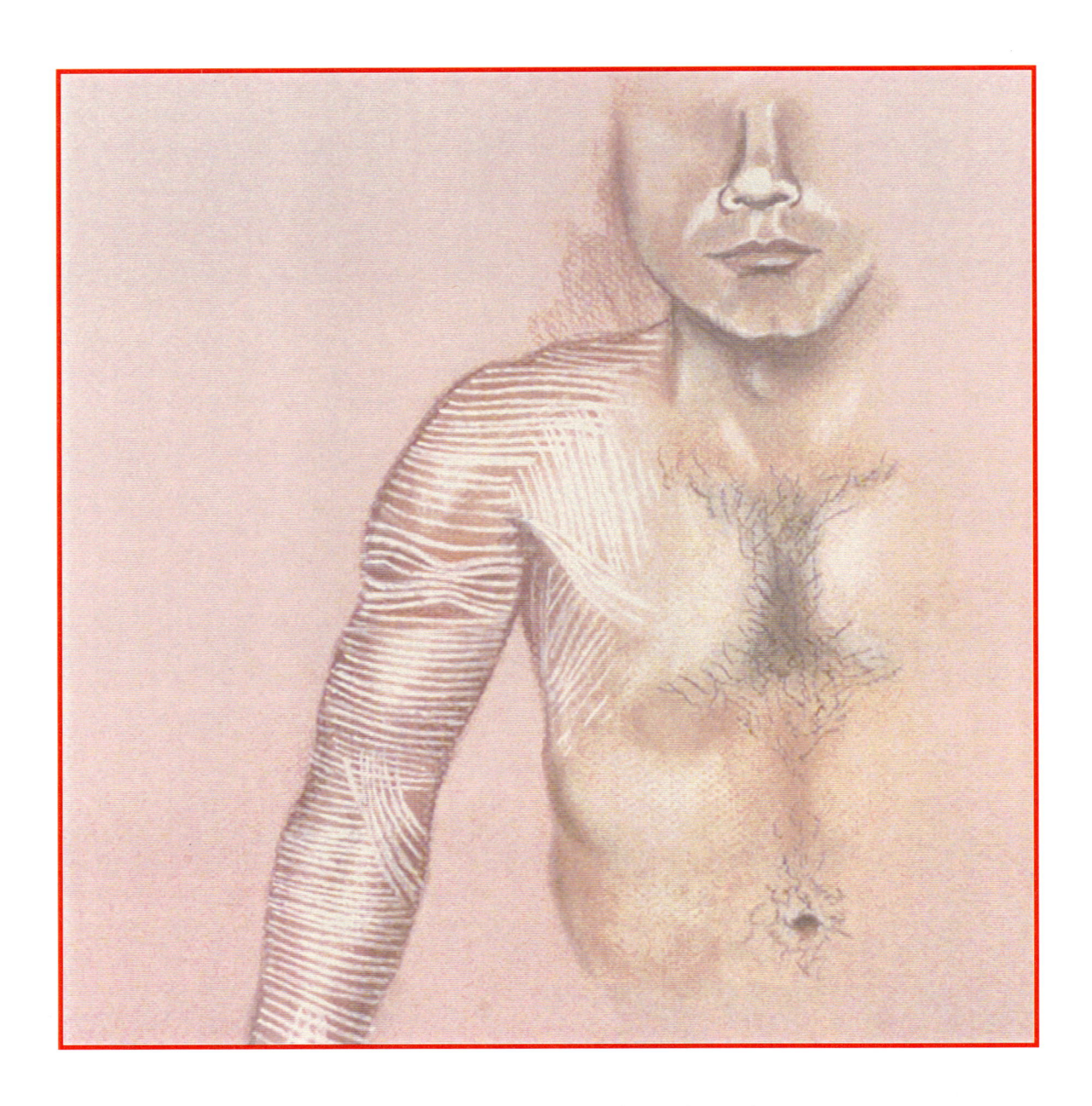

Figure 7-1. Cylinder Distortion of Brachial Fascia

Common manifestations of less symptomatic cylinder injuries include:
- Deep pain in non-jointed areas
- No tenderness to palpation
- Grossly normal motion
- Diffuse or vague discomfort
- Paresthesias
- Spasm

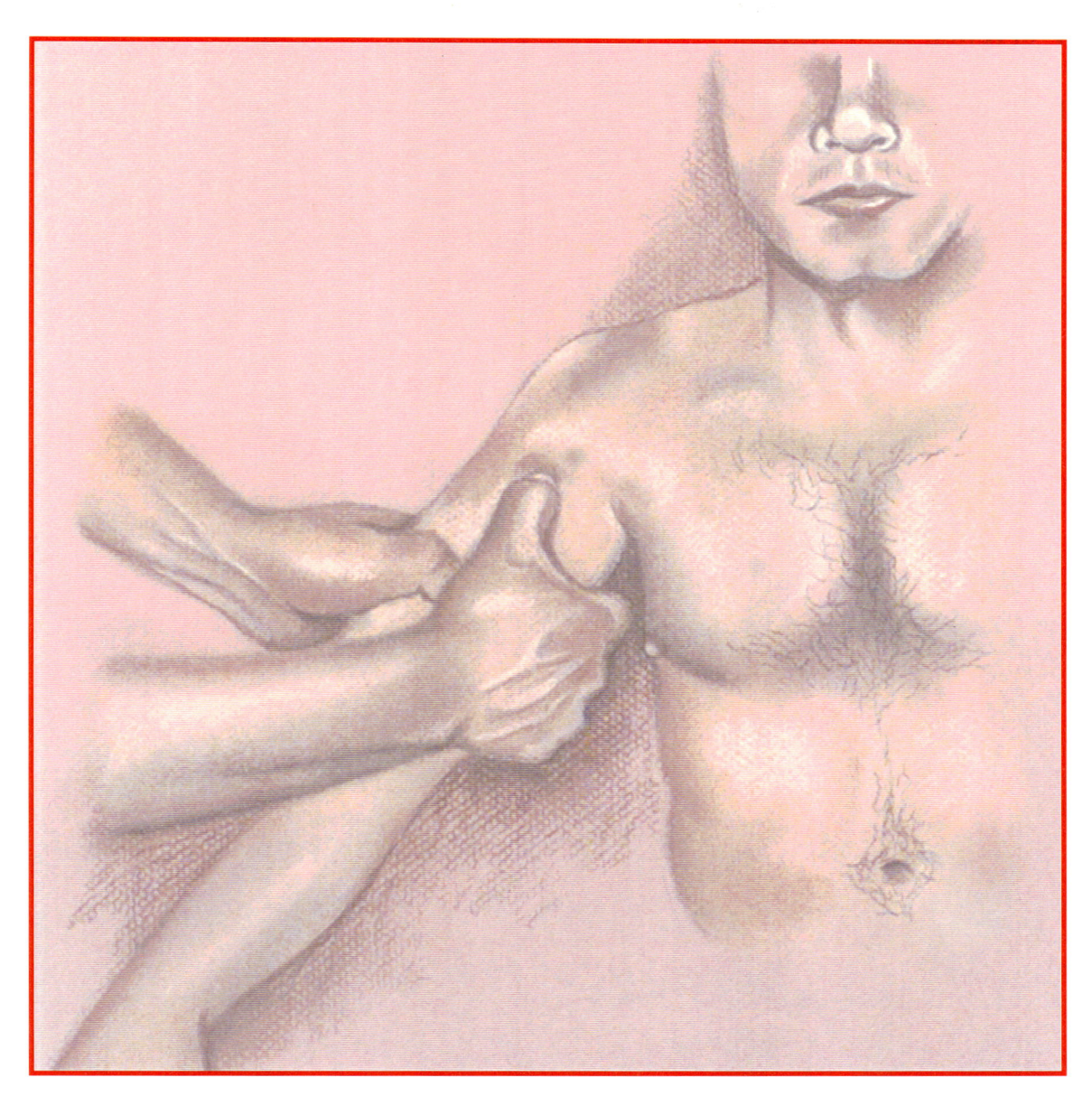

Figure 7-2. Treatment with Double Thumb Cylinder Technique

- Patients attempt to locate the discomfort with their fingers and say something to the effect that, "It's deep in there somewhere, but I can't seem to find it"
- Poor subjective response to muscle relaxers, non-steroidal anti-inflammatory medicines, and narcotic drugs (also true of other fascial distortion types)
- The aching or severe pain may spontaneously abate at the same moment a similar aching or severe pain occurs in an area non-adjacent to the original pain (jumping phenomenon)

CYLINDER TECHNIQUES

In treating cylinder distortions, the goal is to untangle the tangled cylinder coils. This is currently done primarily by one of four techniques:
- Indian burn
- Double thumb
- Squeegee
- Compression cylinder variants

Cylinder distortions can be envisioned as a snarled Slinky® toy, but the tangled coils themselves are so small that they cannot be directly appreciated through palpation. Instead, the tautness of the tissue around them is indicative of their presence.

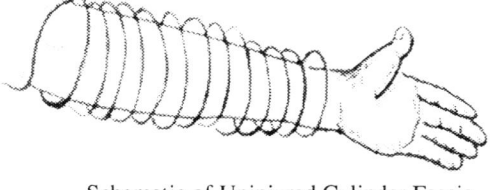

Schematic of Uninjured Cylinder Fascia   Schematic of Distorted Cylinder Fascia

Figure 7-3.

In the *Indian burn* approach, the physician's hands are positioned one to two inches apart and just above and below the symptomatic area. The hands grasp firmly onto and around the involved extremity and pull apart. As traction is maximized, one hand initiates a twisting motion in a clockwise direction while the other hand does so in a counterclockwise direction. The forces of twisting and traction are held until the tautness of the tissue diminishes. If the treatment should be unsuccessful, then reversing the rotation of the hands may be beneficial. The therapy should begin close to the proximal joint and *march down* the extremity by repeating the above sequence over the entire segment of that limb until the distal joint is reached. Failure to march will likely result in an ineffective treatment because the discomfort may *jump* from one area to another. Remember to *never use Indian burn on the upper arm, foot, or ankle* because in those areas the cylinder fascia is very delicate and more cylinder distortions may be created than corrected!

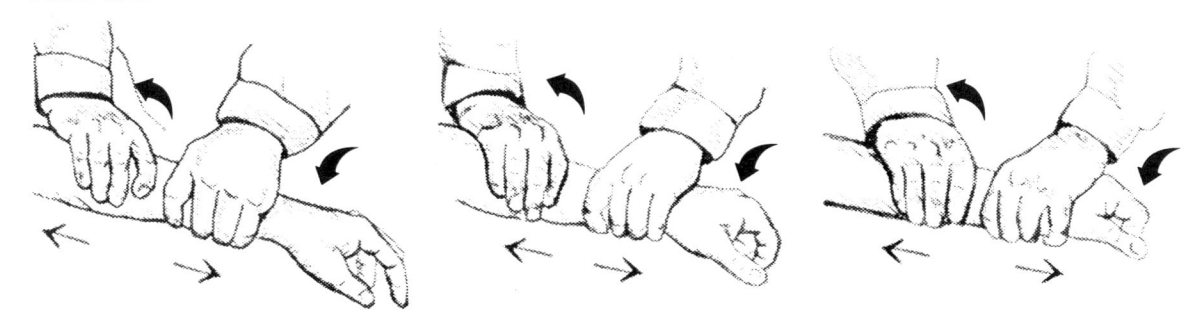

Figure 7-4. Marching Down the Forearm with Indian Burn Cylinder Technique

The *double thumb* approach is designed to correct localized distortions and is far less labor intensive for the physician than is Indian burn cylinder technique. First, the deeper cylinder fascia is treated by applying traction with the thumbs placed to each side of the taut tissue. Since the deeper fibers run parallel to the bone, the direction of force is perpendicular to the axis of the bones. Note that traction is maintained until the release is felt (i.e., the tautness of the tissue diminishes as the coils untangle).

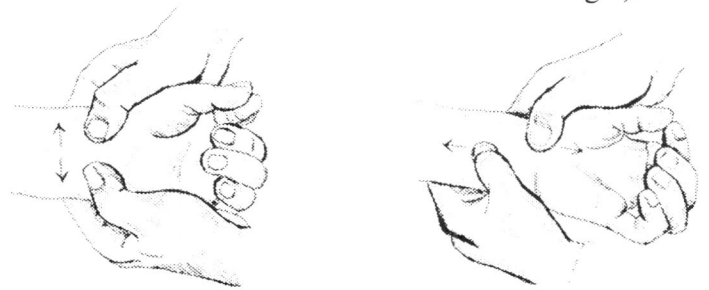

Figure 7-5. Double Thumb Cylinder Technique for Deep (left) and Superficial (right) Layers of Cylinder Fascia

After the deep layer has been corrected, treat the superficial layer. This is done in the same manner, only the direction is changed. To untangle these fibers that encircle the extremity in a perpendicular fashion, traction is applied to the tight tissue so that the force is parallel to the axis of the bones. And just as with the deep layer, force is maintained until the tissue tautness diminishes.

When using the double thumb method, several focal areas may need to be treated, but caution should be exercised so as not to over-treat on any one visit. Also note that with the double thumb approach marching down the limb is unnecessary, instead only symptomatic areas are treated.

The *squeegee technique* is the therapy of choice for those patients with diffuse cylinder pain throughout an entire limb (or a large portion of it). To treat, one or both hands are wrapped around the proximal or distal portion of the extremity and together slide along the limb while a constant squeezing tension is maintained (think of a gas station attendant channeling the water off your windshield with a squeegee wiper).

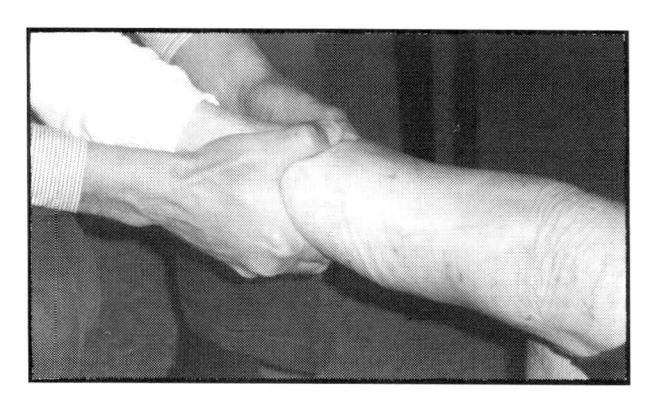

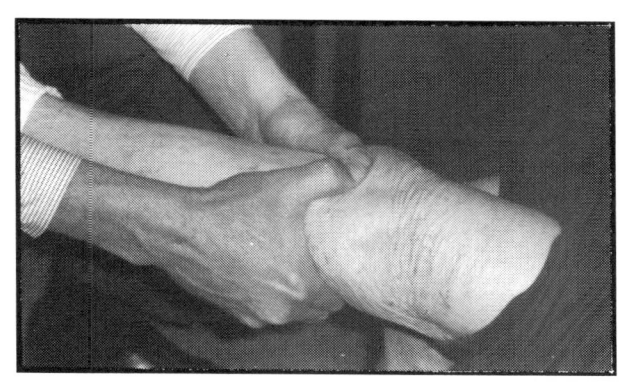

Figure 7-6. Squeegee Cylinder Technique of the Lower Leg

Modifications in cylinder technique in which the fascial coils are pushed together, rather than pulled apart, are possible for all three cylinder techniques (Indian burn, double thumb, and squeegee) and are collectively known as *compression cylinder variants* (CCV). The hand position for double thumb (see Figure 7-7) and Indian burn are identical to what has been shown, but the cylinder fascia is compressed rather than tractioned. In the compression variant for squeegee technique (see Figure 11-7) the hands are placed so that one is positioned at the proximal portion of the affected limb as the other hand grasps the distal limb portion. Together they squeegee the cylinder fascia until they meet in the middle.

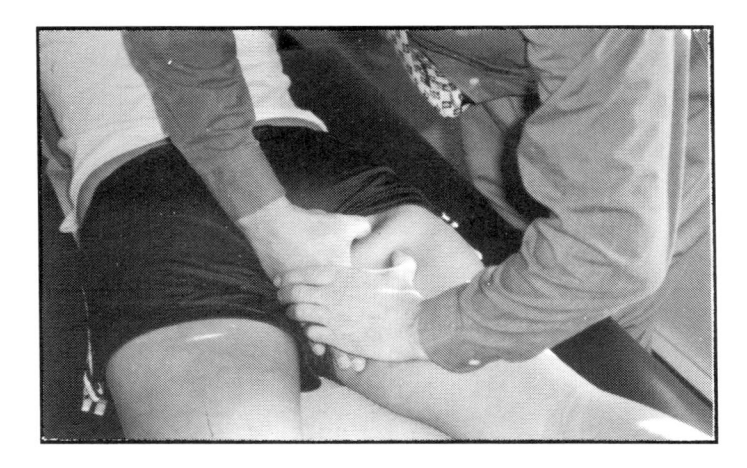

Figure 7-7. Double Thumb Compression Cylinder Variant of the Thigh

Two final thoughts on cylinder distortions: Any pain that jumps from one location to another is always a cylinder distortion; and the comb technique that is used in treating chronic triggerband injuries can also be used in treating chronic cylinder distortions. The reason for this is that the teeth of the comb can help fracture the tiny adhesions that have grown between the overlapping cylinder coils.

Chapter 8

TECTONIC FIXATIONS AND TECTONIC TECHNIQUE

The sixth and most recently described principal fascial distortion type is the tectonic fixation (TF). It is defined as *a physiological alteration in which the fascial surface has lost its ability to properly glide*. And since fixated fascial surfaces can occur in any joint in the body (as well as the viscera), tectonic fixations are common and widespread. Physically the non-gliding surfaces of a tectonic fixation behave almost as if they were two magnets attracting each other. As the name of the distortion implies, these two surfaces jammed together are reminiscent of geological plates of the Earth's crust thrust into one another.

The fixation itself occurs secondary to loss of synovial fluid transport between the two surfaces. With less synovial fluid recycling through the joint, the magnetic field changes and the fascia loses its ability to repel the adjacent tissue or bony surface, and instead attracts it. This *flip-flopping of the magnetic field* is analogous to that of a magnet that when turned over changes from repelling the other magnet to attracting it.

In treating tectonic fixations the goals are:
1. Correct any underlying fascial distortions (particularly triggerbands with adhesions, and refolding distortions)
2. Increase synovial fluid circulation (slow tectonic pump, hot packs, plunger technique)
3. Re-initiate gliding by physically forcing the fixated surfaces to slide (thrusting tectonic techniques such as frogleg and reverse frogleg manipulations, and Kirksville crunch)

Once the stuck structures are budged, some tectonic fixations are instantaneously resolved (this is particularly true of facet TF's), while for more long-standing conditions, multiple treatments are required. In the most severe cases, stagnant synovial fluid degrades from a clear colorless liquid into a thick white paste. In these injuries, resolution occurs only when enough fresh synovial fluid is pumped between the fixated surfaces (and the stagnant fluid is flushed out and reabsorbed) to cause the magnetic field to flip again so that the surfaces once more repel each other.

Three tectonic fixations of primary interest to the general osteopath or orthopedist are:
1. Shoulder
2. Hip
3. Facet

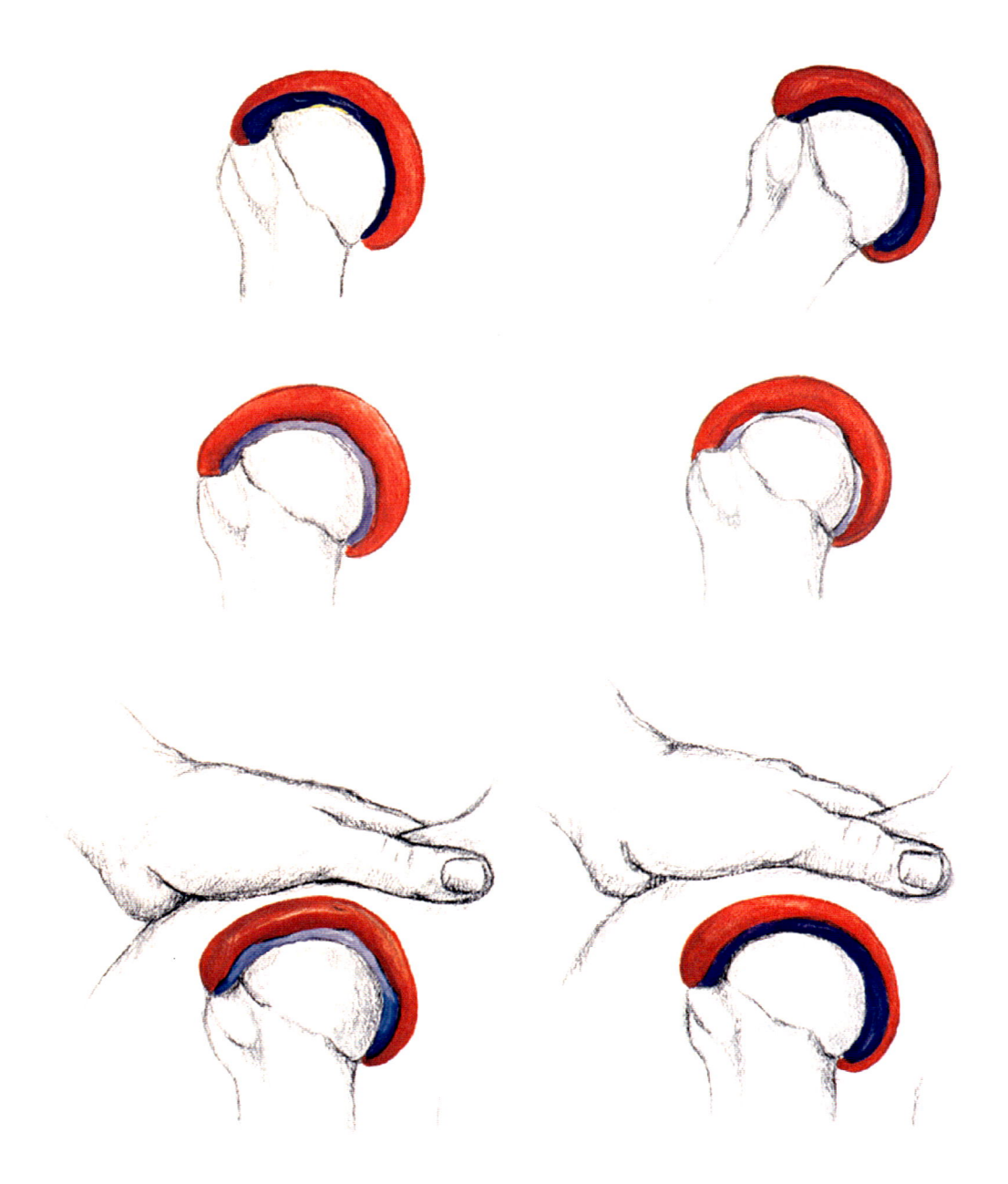

Figure 8-1. Tectonic Fixation of the Shoulder

Top Pictures: With normal shoulder motion the capsule (red) glides on the head of the humerus. This rocking back and forth of the capsule facilitates circulation of synovial fluid (dark blue) within the joint.

Middle Pictures: However, if shoulder motion becomes restricted from an injury, such as a triggerband, the fluid may fail to circulate properly throughout the entire joint. Eventually, small pockets of stagnated fluid accumulate (light blue). In these areas of devitalized synovial fluid, the magnetic field becomes altered so that the capsule and the bone now attract rather than repel each other. When portions of the capsule become fixated on the bone this is called a *tectonic fixation*.

Lower Pictures: Tectonic technique is designed to literally force the capsule to slide. Capsular sliding physically plunges non-stagnant synovial fluid into the fixated areas of the joint and pumps stagnated fluid out where it can be reabsorbed. Once a sufficient quantity of revitalized fluid seeps between the two fixated surfaces, the magnetic field reverts so that the capsule and the bone once again repel each other.

SHOULDER TECTONIC FIXATIONS

In a tectonic fixation of the shoulder, the entire capsule, or a portion of it, has become fixated to the underlying bone (in the orthopedic model, these distortions are commonly classified as adhesive capsulitis). Severely affected patients present with global loss of motion (i.e., diminished or non-existent abduction, external, and internal rotation), and say that they feel as if the joint is a *quart low on oil*. In less severe cases the movement of the shoulder resembles the stiff-jointed *Tin Man* from the movie *The Wizard of Oz*. Note that on physical exam these patients demonstrate an inability to abduct the shoulder without anterior rotation, and can't lay the shoulder flat against the table in the prone swimmers position (see Figure 11-1).

The current preferred treatment of these difficult injuries is:
1. Correct other fascial distortions which generally include
   A. SCHTP
   B. Triggerbands: star, upper trapezius, and anterior and posterior shoulder pathways
   C. Star folding
   D. First-rib refolding
   E. Upper thoracic foldings
   F. Thoracic and cervical facet tectonic fixations
2. Slow tectonic pump of the shoulder
3. Refolding technique of the shoulder
4. Frogleg and reverse frogleg tectonic techniques or other assorted tectonic manipulations

Tectonic Shoulder Techniques

In shoulder tectonic fixations that demonstrate profound loss of motion, slow tectonic pump is a crucial component in the treatment. It is performed with the patient seated or supine and is designed to force fresh synovial fluid between the fixated capsule and humeral head. To treat: Physician grasps the wrist of the affected shoulder with both hands and slowly pumps the extremity by alternately flexing and extending, or abducting and adducting, or tractioning and compressing the shoulder joint (see glossary term *Slow Tectonic Pump*).

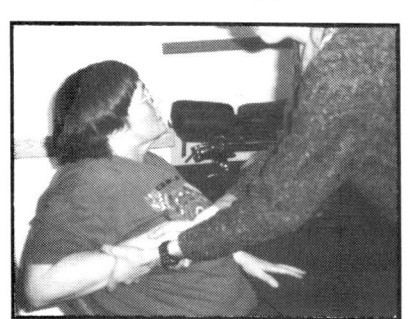

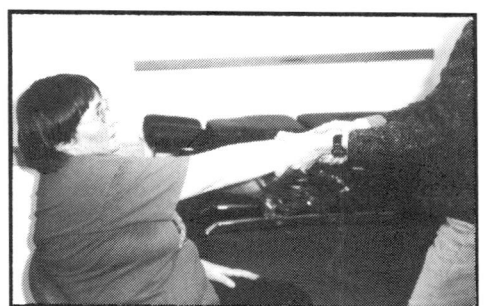

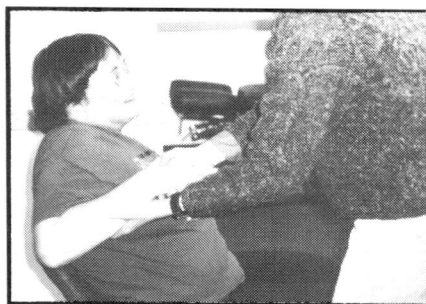

Figure 8-2. Slow Tectonic Pump

Care should be taken to pump the shoulder leisurely (optimal frequency is one cycle every 3-5 seconds) because faster rates don't allow sufficient time for the sluggish devitalized synovial fluid to flow out of the joint. The number of pumping cycles to be employed is determined by:
 1. Degree of fixation
 2. Amount of energy and strength available on the part of the treating orthopath

However, a general rule concerning slow tectonic pump is — *the more the better*.

Frogleg and reverse frogleg manipulations are currently the two most successful thrusting tectonic techniques for the shoulder. In both of these treatments the patient is sitting with the physician standing on the same side as the injured shoulder. Frogleg is performed first, followed by reverse frogleg.

Frogleg technique of right shoulder –
- Physician's right hand grasps right wrist
- Physician's left palm cups right elbow
- Shoulder abducted between 80° and 120°
- Elbow flexed 45°-90°
- Continuous force applied so that elbow is pushed forward as wrist is pulled backward
- Correction is made with a simultaneous quick thrusting of the elbow anteriorly and a swift pulling of the wrist posteriorly

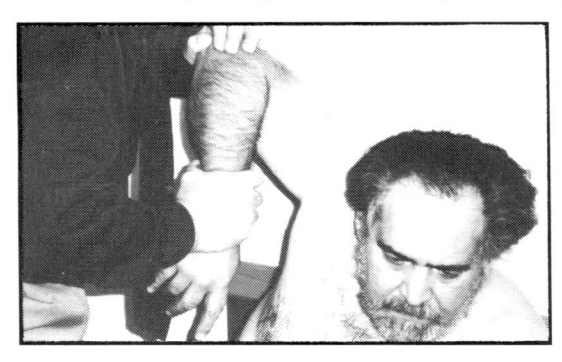

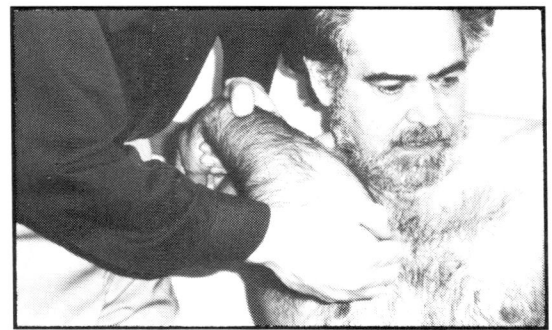

Figure 8-3. Frogleg (left) and Reverse Frogleg (right) Manipulations of the Shoulder

Reverse frogleg technique of right shoulder –
- Physician's right hand cups right elbow
- Physician's left hand grasps right wrist
- Shoulder flexed 60° to 120°
- Elbow fully flexed and pointing forward
- Continuous force applied so that the elbow is pushed toward the opposite shoulder and the wrist is pulled toward the physician
- Correction is made by thrusting the elbow toward the opposite shoulder and pulling the wrist toward the physician

Note that a large pop or slide/clunk accompanies a successful frogleg or reverse frogleg manipulation and that if the two procedures are performed repetitively and slowly they can be used as a form of slow tectonic pump.

Other assorted shoulder tectonic techniques include:
1. Brute force maneuver
2. Whip technique
3. Plunger technique
4. Cupping

The brute force maneuver (see Figure 11-9) is performed with the physician standing behind the patient. The right hand is placed on top of the right shoulder as the left hand is positioned on the left shoulder. The osteopath then leans onto the shoulders from above so that the weight of his or her body is transmitted into the patient's two shoulders. The treating hands are rocked back and forth in a rhythmic fashion to pump synovial fluid by alternating the amount of force directed onto the affected shoulder capsule. Please note that for this procedure to succeed, it is often necessary for the physician to use all of his/her strength and body weight.

The whip technique (see Figure 11-9) is a general shoulder treatment which has the dual role of:
1. Forcing the fixated capsule to slide
2. Correcting unfolding distortions

In this approach, the wrist is held by both of the osteopath's hands while the patient's shoulder and elbow are first fully flexed and then forcefully and suddenly extended. This motion is repeated over and over again in a rapid pace until a desirable outcome is achieved (a pop is heard as the fixated surfaces slide or the contorted fascia unfolds). Note that although the whip technique appears to be a faster and more aggressive form of slow tectonic pump, it is not. This is because the speed of whipping is ineffective in circulating the thickened and stagnated synovial fluid of a long-standing shoulder tectonic fixation.

The plunger technique (see glossary term *Plunger Technique*) is still another tectonic approach in treating particularly stubborn shoulder fixations. In this modality, the mouth of a small sink plunger is suctioned onto the shoulder and pumped 10-20 times before being repositioned. The aim of the procedure is two-fold:
1. Physically force the capsule to slide
2. Pump synovial fluid between the fixated surfaces

A cousin of the plunger technique is cupping. In the modern adaptation of this ancient Chinese custom, a suction gun is utilized to create a vacuum so that glass or plastic bells can be suctioned onto the shoulder (see glossary term *Cupping*). The attached bells influence synovial fluid transport by maintaining a continuous tug on the capsule and fluid. The traction of the capsule pulls it away from the fixated bony surface which allows devitalized joint fluid to escape and fresh fluid to circulate. Patients who are treated with either the plunger or cupping should be forewarned of the obvious but usually harmless side effect of hemorrhagic petechiae (see Figure 9-4).

HIP TECTONIC FIXATIONS

Tectonic fixations of the hip involve the head of the femur and the acetabulum. Although some patients with hip TF's complain of hip or gluteal discomfort, most complain of "low back pain." The associated body language with this distortion is placing the hands over the iliac crests.

Treatment of hip tectonic fixations generally involves only utilizing the hip version of frogleg and reverse frogleg tectonic techniques. However, some stubborn injuries cannot be corrected until the following have been performed:
 1. Triggerband technique of the posterior thigh tightness and lateral thigh pathways
 2. Refolding manipulations of the hip
 3. Slow tectonic pump of the hip

Frogleg technique of the hip is performed with the patient supine and the physician standing beside the table on the same side as the hip to be manipulated. If the right hip is to be treated, the following positioning is required:
- Physician stands on right side of table
- Hip is flexed and externally rotated
- Knee is flexed
- Doctor's right hand grasps the ankle and brings it to midline
- Doctor's left hand is placed on bent knee and pushes inferiorly (i.e., towards foot end of table) as right hand pushes ankle superiorly. Force is increased until barrier is reached
- Thrust is made simultaneously with each hand through the barrier

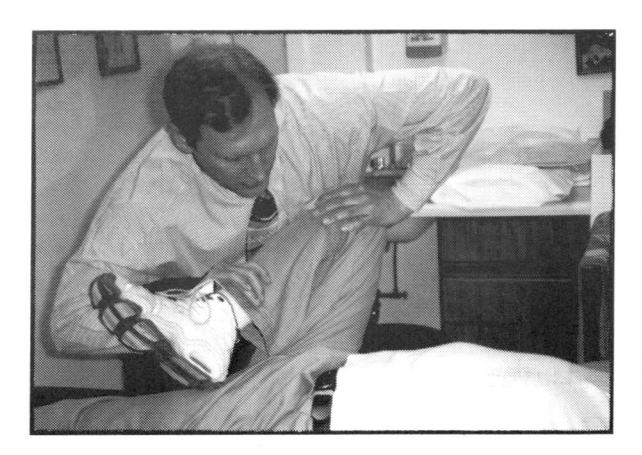

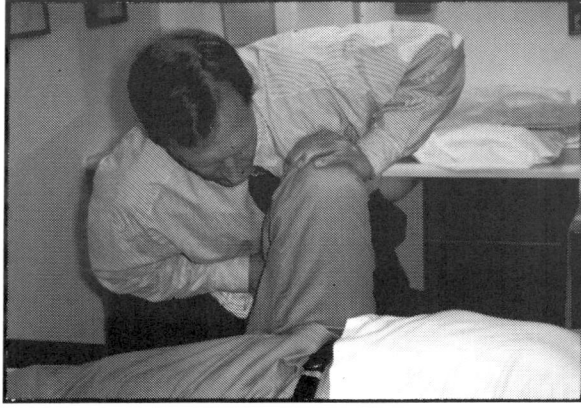

Figure 8-4. Frogleg (left) and Reverse Frogleg (right) Manipulations of the Hip

Reverse frogleg technique is performed immediately following a successful or unsuccessful frogleg treatment. Points to remember in treating the right hip:
- Doctor stands on right side of table
- Doctor's right hand grasps right ankle and pulls it laterally and superiorly
- Doctor's left hand pushes on right knee which is flexed more than 90° – direction of force is both across patient's body and inferiorly
- Force on ankle and knee are increased until barrier is reached, then thrust is made through barrier
- Manipulation is facilitated with compression of hip (leaning chest onto knee)
- In switching from frogleg to reverse frogleg, don't cross the hands or feet
- A successful frogleg or reverse frogleg manipulation is accompanied with an audible slide-clunk or pop

Slow tectonic pump of the hip is performed in much the same manner as it is for the shoulder. One hand grasps the ankle and the other the knee so that the hip and knee can be repetitively flexed and extended, abducted and adducted, and internally and externally rotated. Just as in the shoulder, the optimal speed is one cycle every three to five seconds.

FACET TECTONIC FIXATIONS

Stuck vertebral facet joints are perhaps the most common reason patients seek osteopathic care. The associated verbal assertion that their "back needs to be cracked" is indicative of this particular lesion. Thrusting facet tectonic techniques are in many ways similar to those shown in the folding chapter. The difference is that folding techniques require either traction or compression to engage the paravertebral folding fascia, whereas tectonic techniques are dependent upon neutral direction thrusts to focus the force into the facet joints.

Examples of facet tectonic techniques include:
- Cervical – sitting or supine neutral thrust
- Thoracic – Kirksville crunch (a.k.a. dog technique), double pisiform thrust, chair neutral thrust
- Lumbar – lumbar roll, chair neutral thrust

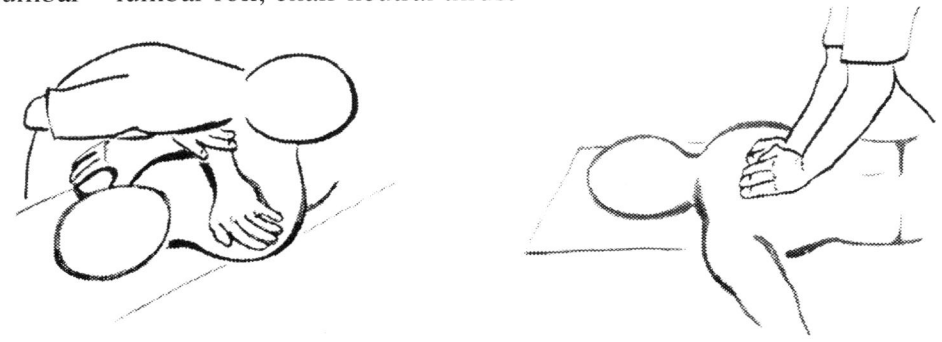

Figure 8-5. Kirksville Crunch (left) and Double Pisiform Thrust (right)

TECTONIC FIXATIONS AND HEAT

Unlike the other five principal fascial distortions, tectonic fixations clinically respond favorably to the application of a hot, wet compress prior to treatment with tectonic techniques. The reason for this is that heat seems to temporarily (and minimally) decrease the thickness of the synovial fluid which allows for improved joint fluid circulation. However, it should be strongly noted that heat has a tendency to make any accompanying acute triggerbands, herniated triggerpoints, continuum distortions, folding distortions, or cylinder distortions considerably more symptomatic and clinically more difficult to correct.

Chapter 9

SYNOPSIS OF SELECTED FASCIAL DISTORTION CONCEPTS

ORTHOPEDIC CONSIDERATIONS

Orthopedic treatments can be thought of as forms of fascial distortion techniques. Examples: Reduction of a dislocation is a generalized folding technique, the surgical repair of a ruptured quadriceps tendon includes pulling and untwisting the fibers (triggerband technique), and carpal tunnel release surgery involves an incision of the retinaculum (fracturing adhesions and cutting apart tangled cylinder coils).

When orthopedic injuries are consciously envisioned as fascial distortions, specific modifications in orthopedic procedures can be made. For instance, in the reduction of a dislocation, if the goal is to unfold the fascia, then the added finesse of doing so allows for an easier reduction and minimizes pharmaceutical support. And in the case of a quadriceps rupture, if the remaining distorted fascial bands are intrasurgically straightened, post-operative stiffness is reduced. Similarly, if carpal tunnel surgery were focused on selectively untangling cylinder distortions and ironing out distorted fascial fibers, the surgery itself would be less intrusive than it currently is and much more effective.

Orthopathically, bone fractures are perceived to be extensions of fascial distortions into the osseous matrix. Spiral fractures, for instance, follow the pathway of a single fascial triggerband into the bone as it becomes a *bony triggerband*. Chip and avulsion fractures result when the challenged transition zone is unable to shift quickly enough into its proper protective configuration (osseous if the force is unidirectional and ligamentous if it is multidirectional). And finally, comminuted fractures occur when a fascial or ligamental triggerband is driven into a continuum distortion and the bony matrix is splintered (this is analogous to a block of ice being shattered by an ice pick).

In fractures of the forearm, wrist, ankle, and leg, orthopedic management (either intrasurgically or pre- or post-casting) could include correction of interosseous membrane folding distortions (see Figure 9-1). The realigned and properly functioning membrane would then hold the fractured fragments of the bone in closer proximity, thereby accelerating healing, decreasing casting time, and lessening the chance of creating a tectonic fixation. And since there would be few, if any, folding distortions after removal of the cast, normal range of motion would be expected.

Figure 9-1. Road Map Analogy and Forearm Fracture

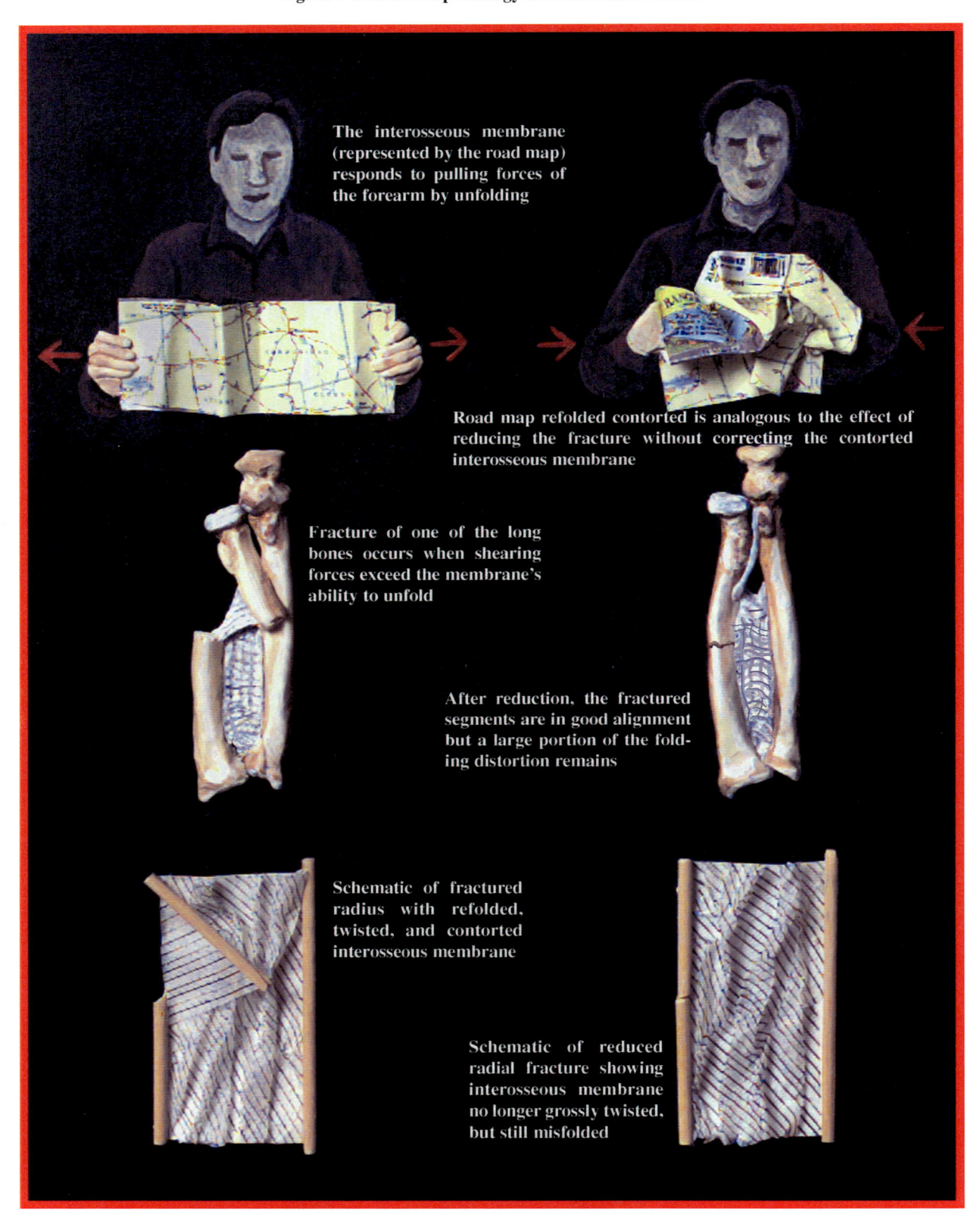

The interosseous membrane (represented by the road map) responds to pulling forces of the forearm by unfolding

Road map refolded contorted is analogous to the effect of reducing the fracture without correcting the contorted interosseous membrane

Fracture of one of the long bones occurs when shearing forces exceed the membrane's ability to unfold

After reduction, the fractured segments are in good alignment but a large portion of the folding distortion remains

Schematic of fractured radius with refolded, twisted, and contorted interosseous membrane

Schematic of reduced radial fracture showing interosseous membrane no longer grossly twisted, but still misfolded

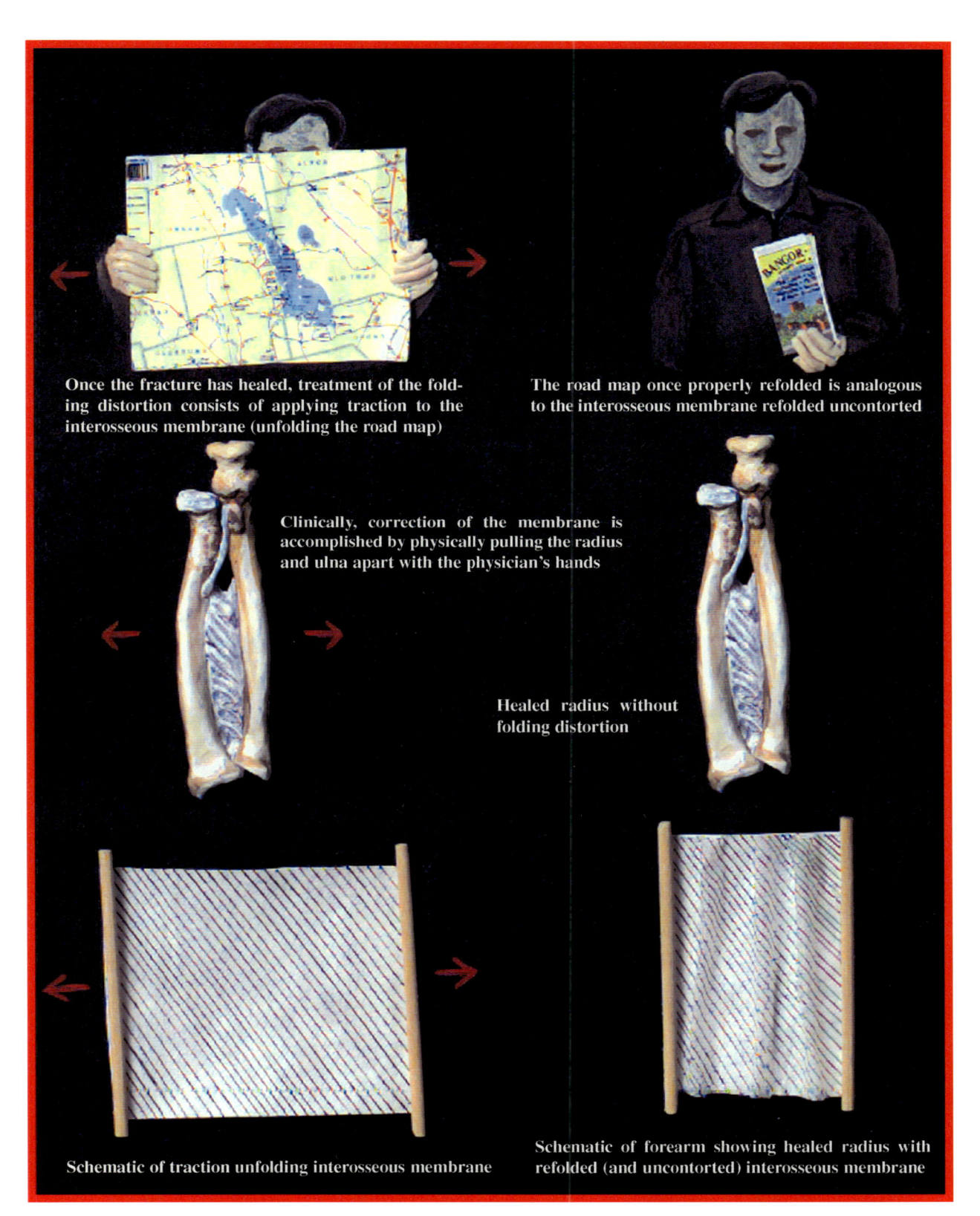

Once the fracture has healed, treatment of the folding distortion consists of applying traction to the interosseous membrane (unfolding the road map)

The road map once properly refolded is analogous to the interosseous membrane refolded uncontorted

Clinically, correction of the membrane is accomplished by physically pulling the radius and ulna apart with the physician's hands

Healed radius without folding distortion

Schematic of traction unfolding interosseous membrane

Schematic of forearm showing healed radius with refolded (and uncontorted) interosseous membrane

The success of any specific orthopedic intervention is, at least in part, contingent upon the type of fascial distortion present. For instance, injecting a frozen shoulder with a steroid is only likely to be effective in a tectonic fixation. Orthopathically, the positive outcome from the drug itself is thought to be derived from the increased volume and improved synovial fluid circulation which occurs as the added liquid is physically pumped into the joint. Then over the next several hours or days, the now re-circulating fluid slowly seeps between the fixated surfaces and changes the magnetic field, which allows for capsular sliding. In the future, more specific drugs or solutions could be developed which would be even more successful.* And perhaps the best treatment to come will be drawing synovial fluid from another joint and injecting and pumping it back and forth through the fixated joint.

In addition to volume enhancement, steroid injections (and prescriptions) have the physiological effect of chemically shifting the entire continuum of musculoskeletal tissues so that osseous components are pulled from the bone into the attaching fascial structures. The efficacy of this approach can be seen in treating a specific condition such as tendonitis. In the FDM, the underlying anatomical injuries associated with the symptoms clinically diagnosed as tendonitis are triggerbands or continuum distortions.

In the case of triggerband tendonitis, the sensation of pain is due not only to the mechanical shortening of the fibers but also to the sensory changes secondary to altered fluid transmission in the osseous-depleted portions of the fiber that are distal to the twist (*roadblock effect*). The subjective benefit of steroid treatment is that the shifting of osseous components into the fascia floods and replenishes the ligamental fibers and thereby eliminates one of the pain-generating mechanisms of the anatomical injury. In the case of continuum tendonitis, the flood of osseous components through the transition zone forces the entire zone into the osseous configuration. Having all of the areas of the zone in one configuration balances the mechanical tension forces and thereby eliminates the dichotomy of sensory tension that is subjectively appreciated as pain.

However, as the physiological effects from the steroid diminish over time, the flow of osseous components into the fascia from the bone slows and then reverses. In the triggerband this means that areas distal to the twist once again experience deficiencies in osseous components. In the case of tendonitis from a continuum distortion, the transition zone slowly shifts back into the neutral state, but if the portion of the zone that was stuck in the osseous configuration remains stuck, the continuum distortion seems to reoccur. In either of these two scenarios, patients are likely to express the renewal of their symptoms by saying "the shot wore off."

Other desired effects and side effects of steroid therapy involve this same shifting process of the continuum. The apparent increased muscular strength is derived from osseous components stiffening the myofascia and providing a firmer background for muscular contractions. The ligaments, like the tendons, become less flexible and more brittle, making them susceptible to tears between the fibers (i.e., forming triggerbands). And the

---

*Newly introduced viscosupplementation injectables include Hylan G-F 20 and Sodium Hyaluronate.

bone itself becomes osteoporotic which increases the risk of unidirectional forces causing compression and stress fractures.

Although steroids are the most common chemical therapy for manipulating the musculoskeletal continuum, other non-drug approaches also exist. Two examples of structural continuum technique are orthopedic pinning/tractioning for lengthening long bones, and the application of orthodontic braces. As we look to the new millennium, the next level of orthopedic care will likely center on understanding and controlling the continuum process.

THE GENERATION OF FASCIAL DISTORTIONS FROM PRE-EXISTING INJURIES

Fascial distortions not only occur from injuries, but can arise from other pre-existing fascial distortions. For example, if a continuum sprained ankle is left untreated, a triggerband may form. The triggerband occurs because the more osseous portion of the transition zone (i.e., the portion inhabited by the continuum distortion) is functionally stiffer and thus responds differently to extrinsic forces than the non-injured portion. Over time, the more brittle osseous fibers tear apart from the more flexible fibers . . . and thus a triggerband is born.

The reverse process also occurs (i.e., continuum distortions are formed from triggerbands). In a triggerband sprained ankle, the twisted fibers are functionally shorter and exert more tension on the transition zone. Eventually that portion of the zone shifts into the more osseous configuration . . . and thus a continuum distortion is born.

THE PHYSIOLOGICAL EFFECT OF A TRIGGERBAND IN A LIGAMENT

In the fascial distortion model, a ligamental triggerband acts as a roadblock of fluid transport flowing between the two bones bridged by the ligament. The bone on one side of the triggerband becomes deprived of normal osseous material while the other side is saddled with a surplus that eventually overflows into the periosteum, fascia, and the ligament itself. Over time this imbalance becomes radiographically evident as both a relative osteoporosis (the bone with decreased osseous flow) and as degenerative changes of the joint surface of the bone saturated with osseous flow. This relationship of osteoporosis and osteoarthritis is considered within the FDM to be a functional one in which these two disorders are viewed as being physiological mirror images of each other.

VISUALIZING A LIGAMENTAL TRIGGERBAND

One way to envision ligamental triggerbands is to think of them as being comprised of fascial fibers stuck in the wavy configuration (see Figure 9-2). In the unloaded condition, when the muscle is resting and the ligament isn't performing work, knee ligamental fibers are wavy. In the loaded condition, when the muscle is contracting and the ligament is working, they are straight. But when an uneven force is applied, the crosslinks which bundle the fibers together become fractured, and the unloaded fibers tear apart and

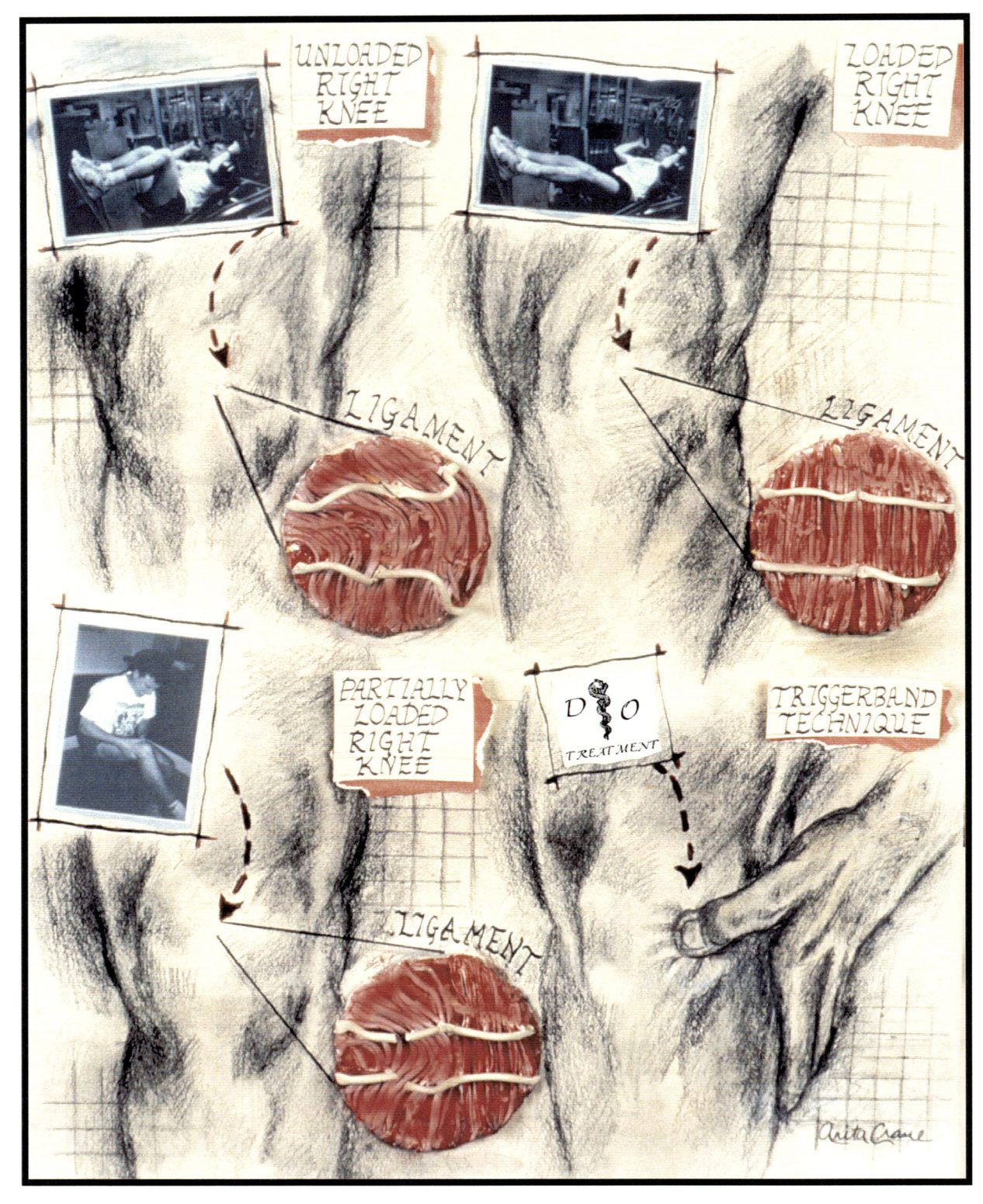

Figure 9-2. Ligamental Triggerband

Unloaded ligamental fibers are wavy (upper left) and loaded fibers are straight (upper right). If the ligament is torqued during either loading or unloading, some of the crosslinks may fracture. This causes the non-bundled fibers to become stuck in the wavy configuration (bottom left). Triggerband technique (bottom right) irons out the wave, re-approximates the parallel fibers, and realigns the crosslinks.

become separated from the loaded fibers. Since the separated fibers are no longer properly attached, they don't straighten when loaded and are therefore incapable of performing work. Clinically, the more fibers involved, the weaker and more painful the ligament becomes.

Triggerband technique is designed to *unstick* these stuck fibers by ironing out the wave and re-approximating the tear. Once the fibers are repositioned, the crosslinks instantly reattach. The anatomical restoration of the injured fibers not only eliminates the pain, it reverses the pathology. The corrected ligament not only feels better, but has normal strength, motion, and flexibility.

LIGAMENTAL/TENDON TEARS

Although MRI evaluation and surgical inspection of severe sprains often reveal a tear across the width of the ligament or tendon, in the FDM this anatomical injury is considered to be a collection of longitudinally separated fibers. Tears occur in the following steps:
1. Repetitive injurious motions focus forces into specific portions of ligament or tendon which sequentially rip individual fibers apart (triggerbands form).
2. The aggregation of longitudinally separated fibers span the width of the ligament or tendon (may be seen on MRI and interpreted as a partial tear).
3. Since the fibers of the ligament or tendon can no longer collectively absorb injurious forces, the separated fibers tear one by one until a single physical activity (such as pushing a lawn mower) suddenly causes the remaining intact fibers to also lacerate. The *straw that broke the camel's back* gives the patient the impression that this terminal event was solely responsible for the ligament or tendon tearing.

Figure 9-3. Achilles Tendon Tear
Longitudinally twisted and thus separated fibers of an injured Achilles tendon (middle drawing)
diminish the strength of the tendon and allow for horizontal tears (right drawing)

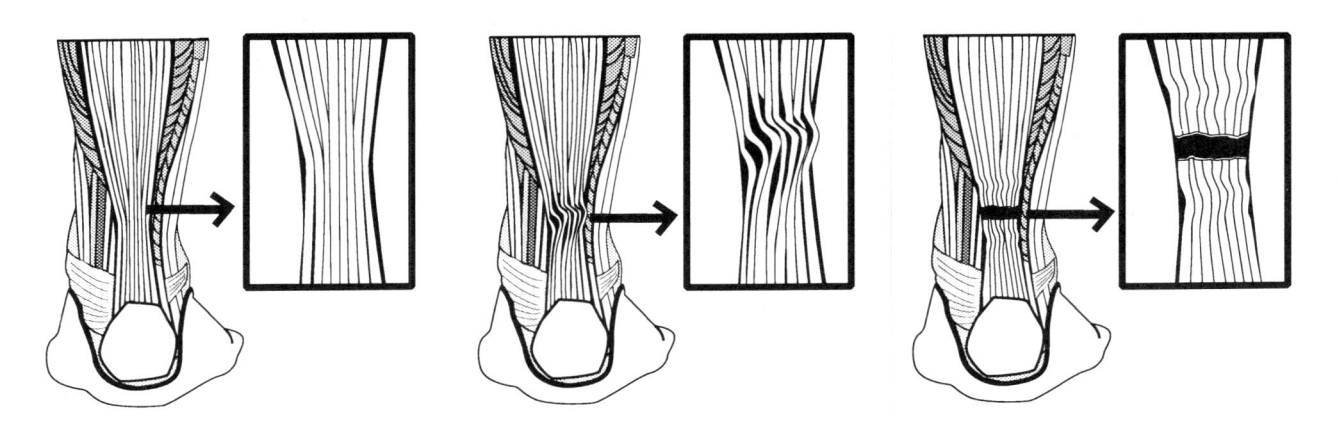

Normal Achilles Tendon   Triggerbands Form Across Tendon   Tendon Tear

PREDICTING SPORTS INJURIES AND ENHANCING ATHLETIC PERFORMANCE

Although the bulk of this book is focused on the treatment of musculoskeletal injuries, the fascial distortion model has another important application — to predict and prevent injuries before they happen. In this aspect, the FDM is a valuable tool in sports medicine to assist athletes, physicians, and trainers in determining who is likely to be injured and why. Orthopathic techniques can then be used to correct the injury before it becomes symptomatic.

The first step in predicting future injuries is to review the past history of the person in question. If he or she sustained a strain, pulled muscle, or sore shoulder that had to be *worked through*, or *got better over time*, this indicates that an unresolved fascial distortion is present. Although the athlete may be performing at what appears to be an acceptable level, this same history suggests that an underlying fascial distortion exists which is restricting potential. Correcting the distortion not only avoids future injury, it also enhances current performance. An example of this can be seen in a baseball pitcher who in the past complained of a sore arm or shoulder. He may have had to avoid throwing for several weeks until he could do so again without pain. The fact that he says his arm "feels fine" does not mean that it is. Even though he has no current complaints, he is still injured because the distortion that caused his disability has never been corrected. He is, therefore, a *walking time bomb* for a future problem.

In predicting a future extremity injury, motion should be carefully examined. If the shoulder of a baseball pitcher, for instance, demonstrates loss of internal rotation (gross loss of total height or even subtle changes, such as decrease in speed or loss of hand rotation, see Figures 11-2 and 11-3), the player should be treated as soon as possible. Ignoring the distortion will result in unnecessary pain, sub-optimal athletic performance, and recurring injuries. Once properly treated, the athlete should be able to throw harder, longer, and more accurately than before. His additional bonus is a decrease in the likelihood of a serious injury. The same enhancement in performance is possible for sprinters, runners, football players, ballerinas, golfers, basketball players, and in fact athletes of every kind. The significance of fascial distortions in athletic performance cannot be emphasized enough. For instance, if a world-class sprinter should have just one small triggerband in his or her hamstring, this may be the competitive difference between finishing first and fifth.

ORTHOPATHIC INTERPRETATION OF CHRONIC PAIN

The orthopedic concept of *chronic* is contingent on time; if an injury has been present for six months or a year, then it is considered to be chronic. This temporal perspective implies that chronic injuries are long-standing (or even permanent), but says nothing about the nature of the anatomical injury, or why such injuries have failed to heal. In the fascial distortion model, chronic pain is viewed from an anatomical perspective. Once fascial adhesions form, the injury becomes chronic. Since fascial distortions of any kind can eventually generate triggerbands, and since adhesions form from the torn crosslinks of triggerbands, any fascial injury can become chronic. Note that splinting or resting injuries tends to increase fascial adhesion formation because the muscular movements which fracture healing mis-attached fibers are minimized. Therefore, to prevent injuries from becoming chronic, triggerbands need to be corrected before adhesions form. Physical activities such as stretching and exercising are also useful since they help realign separated fascial fibers and keep crosslinks from inappropriately attaching to adjacent structures.

From a clinical perspective, identifying chronic pain patients is not difficult; these people have multiple areas of restricted motion in more than one plane and direction. On palpation the fascial structures are tight and are pulled from above, below, and beside the primary distortion. And unlike acute pain patients who define their discomfort clearly, chronic pain patients generalize, "It hurts everywhere," or "It just hurts." This inability to differentiate the pain into simple categories such as *sharp*, *tight*, *dull*, *ache*, or *tender* is a fundamental clinical characteristic of chronic pain syndrome which is often mistaken for malingering. With the FDM, it is not difficult to understand why those with acute injuries are more precise in their descriptions. They have only one or several small anatomical distortions to decipher. But chronic pain patients have multiple distortions and multiple distortion types to describe. Compounding the problem is the fact that adhesions have tied all of these distortions together into a confusing hodgepodge of pathological disarray. Just when a pull is felt in one direction, his/her brain receives simultaneous input of an ache, a sharp pain, and a dull pain, etc. Although these individuals may attempt to describe where and how they hurt, they often can't.

TREATING CHRONIC PAIN WITH FASCIAL DISTORTION TECHNIQUES

The rationale in using fascial distortion techniques is simple: First make the injury acute again and then correct the acute injury. Making the injury acute is done by simply breaking the adhesions. Once the adhesions are broken the injury is no longer considered chronic, and thus is no longer incurable. Breaking the adhesions is done with aggressive triggerband technique. Often maximum force is used as the distorted fascial fibers are re-aligned and the adhesions are *plowed through*. As the adhesions are broken, most patients with folding distortions or tectonic fixations will say something to the effect that the treated area "feels like it needs to pop." This is the *green light* for using thrusting manipulation. When this occurs, a patient who was very difficult to manipulate before triggerband technique, now becomes easy to manipulate. The same person who refused manipulation in the past may now be asking that it be done. This is a favorable indication that the chronic injury has been made acute, and that the acute injury is being properly treated.

Since the fracturing of adhesions is traumatizing to the fascial structures, bruising may occur. In addition, there is typically soreness lasting several days. For this reason, three to four days between the first and second treatments are allowed for the tissues to recuperate. One day less down time is usually needed between the second and third, and one day less than that between the third and fourth treatments. In contrast, acute pain patients can be treated again the very next day.

After two or three aggressive sessions, the treatments become less than half as painful, down time between sessions is only a day or two, and surprisingly, little or no bruising occurs no matter how much force is used. As the injury resolves, motion improves, tightness decreases, and pain begins to feel similar to when the injury first happened.

Note that some chronic pain patients present initially with cylinder distortions. This is because the torn fascial band crosslinks have adhered to the superficial cylindric fascial coils and caused them to tangle. Treatment of chronic cylinder distortions includes not only triggerband technique, but the comb technique, which both separates the tangled fibers and fractures the adhesions. In the comb technique, a steel grooming comb is raked over the affected area every day or two for four to eight sessions. Despite the somewhat menacing appearance of the instrument, it is typically only uncomfortable for the first one or two treatments.

FINESSE AND BRAWN OF FASCIAL DISTORTION TECHNIQUES

In the FDM, finesse and brawn are concepts of clinical practicality. Finesse is the ability to modify the precise actions of a manipulative technique so that it can be specifically applied to each individual injury. Brawn, in contrast, means that the necessary and appropriate amount of physical force is utilized to make the anatomical correction. As a whole, manipulative fascial distortion techniques tend to be both more exact and more aggressive than other osteopathic therapies and, from a purely mechanical point of view, can be classified as either thumb or whole hand treatments. The breakdown is shown below:

Thumb	Whole Hand
Triggerband technique	Folding technique
Herniated triggerpoint therapy	Cylinder technique
Continuum technique	(Indian burn/squeegee)
Cylinder technique (double thumb)	Tectonic technique

Thumb Techniques

In orthopathic medicine, the human thumb is appreciated as an instrument of great manipulative dexterity. It is the ideal tool for pushing, shoving, and moving small structures such as fascial distortions. It is compact and strong, tactile and flexible. And unlike the fingers, it bends only once in its middle which allows the treating force to be focused evenly and precisely beneath it.

In all FDM thumb techniques, the initial position of the thumb is essentially the same. The thumb metacarpophalangeal joint is held in a slightly abducted posture as the interphalangeal joint is flexed. The fingers are used to steady the hand and are stretched apart from the thumb. The hand itself is held loosely so that the wrist can be rotated to the appropriate angle. Direction of force is through the distal phalanx of the thumb. For this reason, the forearm, wrist, and thumb should not be in a straight line. If that is the case, the thumb is forced into extension (and ultimately hyperextension) which displaces the focus of contact from the tip of the thumb to the volar aspect (i.e., where a thumbprint is obtained). This widens the contact surface, unsteadies the force, and decreases endurance.

To be successful with thumb techniques, the contact point must be just slightly to the volar aspect of the end of the distal tuft. This is particularly true in treating small triggerbands and in all continuum distortions. To help steady the treating hand, the non-treating hand and thumb may grip around the treating hand or thumb to help direct the force. Please note that to ensure patient comfort the treating thumbnail should be kept as short as possible.

In treating large herniated triggerpoints, a widened surface of the thumb (more of the volar aspect) is used. Since HTP's tend to be moderate to large in size and fairly soft, this wider surface is necessary. As the HTP begins to release, constant force is maintained. Near the end of release, the thumb-tip is slightly extended and the volar aspect is gently rocked back and forth. This final act of herniated triggerpoint therapy is called *milking* and helps draw the protruded tissue below the fascial plane.

In continuum technique the release is much smaller and faster than in herniated triggerpoint therapy. However, at the instant of release, it is helpful to increase the amount of force by again extending the thumb. This slight increase in pressure directly into the shifting transition zone can also be thought of as milking the release.

Thumb cylinder techniques (double thumb and double thumb CCV) are best utilized in the treatment of focal cylinder distortions. They are perhaps the easiest of all the FDM techniques to master. However, their one major drawback is their inability to combat the *jumping phenomenon* which in some patients can be annoying, irritating, and confusing all at once. Note that when jumping occurs, whole hand cylinder techniques are the preferred approach.

Thumb Strength/Size

Although the human thumb is a wonderful instrument of medical precision, it has limitations. When FDM techniques — particularly triggerband technique — are first being learned, there is often an accompanying degree of thumb fatigue and soreness. Fortunately, with time and practice, strength and stamina improve markedly! Some osteopaths erroneously believe that they will never acquire the appropriate strength to effectively perform triggerband technique because their thumbs are too small. What these small-thumbed physicians may not realize is that for what they may lack in size, they make up for in precision. A small tip is easier to *worm* through tissue layers because it has less bulk and drag. Also it can maintain a much narrower focus on the distortion than a thick thumb can. And in certain areas such as the face and hands, small treating thumbs are advantageous.

Whole Hand Techniques

Most folding, cylinder, and tectonic treatments require both treating hands. All these therapies necessitate some amount of brute strength (particularly in long-standing injuries) and in some ways demand more effort than thumb techniques. As discussed earlier, folding technique is either a modified traction or compression therapy which requires upper arm strength and stamina to be successful. However, the more precise the technique the less physical force is necessary to make the correction. For example, in the treatment of a long-standing injury, such as a frozen wrist secondary to fracture, the finesse involved consists of:

1. Envisioning the injury as a folding distortion of the radial-ulna interosseous membrane
2. Making folding/thrusting manipulations that are anatomically directed (i.e., forcefully thrusting one of the bones away from or into the other bone at a 45° angle)*

Whole hand cylinder techniques (squeegee, Indian burn and their CCV counterparts) are treatments of choice for cylinder distortions that involve large segments or areas of the thorax or limbs. And although to the onlooker these therapies appear effortless, nothing could be further from the truth! Both Indian burn and squeegee, at times, tax the strength of the treating hands and forearms to their limits.

Tectonic techniques engage tectonic fixations either directly (by using both hands to shove the capsule) or indirectly (by using the limb as a lever). Note that indirect approaches (frogleg and reverse frogleg manipulations) require predominantly finesse, whereas direct approaches (such as brute force maneuvers) necessitate the use of copious amounts of brawn.

Practice Makes Perfect

Although both finesse and brawn are important components of a successful treatment, there is no substitute for good old-fashioned practice. Arnold Palmer verbalized this in explaining his success. "The funny thing about golf," he said, "is the more I practice, the luckier I get."

---

*Note that in manipulating the radial-ulna interosseous membrane the inclination of the osteopath is to traction/thrust one of the bones apart from the other at a 90° angle. Although the 90° traction/thrust hand placement is more comfortable than it is for the 45° treatment, the 90° approach is rarely successful. Reason: The preponderance of fibers of the folding fascia that become injured in a fracture are those that cross obliquely from the radius to the ulna rather than at right angles to the bones.

SIDE EFFECTS, CONTRAINDICATIONS, HEAT, AND ICE

The most common side effect of FDM techniques is pain during treatment (close to 100 percent of the time with triggerband and continuum techniques and herniated triggerpoint therapy, less so in cylinder, folding, and tectonic techniques). Erythema of the skin also occurs with triggerband and comb techniques. Soreness and tenderness following FDM treatments are variable. Some patients are quite sore for several days, others are not. Bruising occurs most frequently from the first several chronic pain treatments and is temporary. Hemorrhagic petechiae are expected with use of plunger technique and cupping.

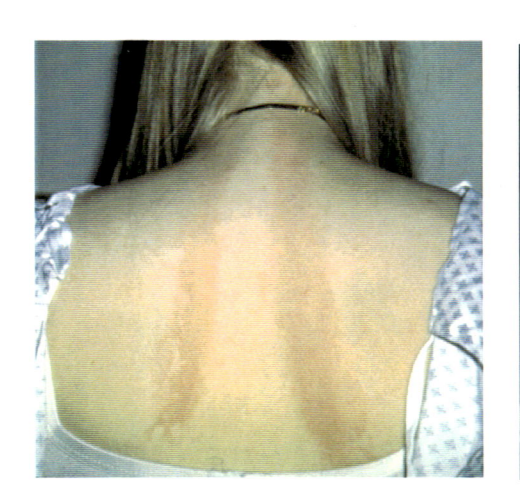

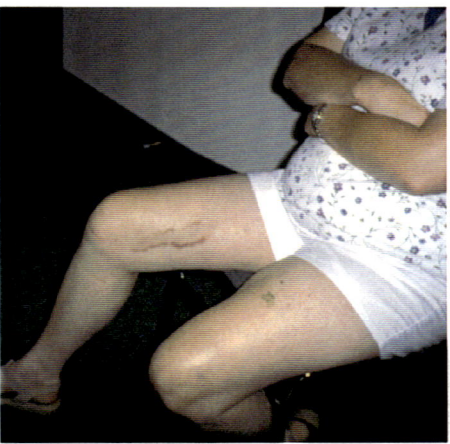

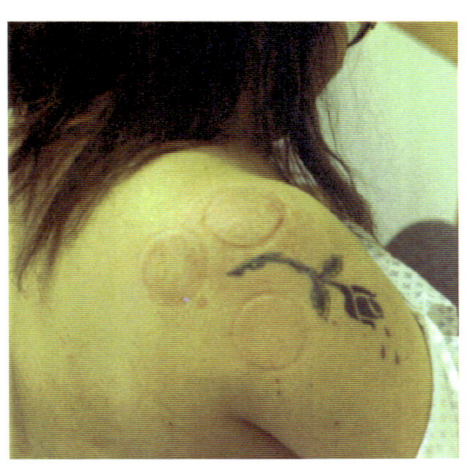

Figure 9-4. Erythema, Bruising, and Hemorrhagic Petechiae

Although undesirable reactions from treatments are possible, FDM techniques, when properly applied, have a very low rate of adverse effects. Still, complications could occur and be anything from stroke to phlebitis. Each physician should decide what he or she feels comfortable treating with each individual patient. Contraindications to FDM techniques are mostly relative and a partial list is offered. Each doctor should, of course, use his or her best judgment before employing these (or any other) treatment modalities.

Partial List of Contraindications

Aneurysms	Open wounds
Arteriosclerosis	Osteomyelitis
Bleeding disorders	Phlebitis
Bone fractures	Poor doctor/patient rapport
Cancer	
Cellulitis	Pregnancy (treatment of abdomen or pelvis)
Collagen vascular diseases	
Edema	Previous strokes
Hematomas	Skin wounds
Infections	Vascular diseases
Infectious arthritis	

Vasovagal responses such as nausea, dizziness, fainting, and vomiting rarely occur. Note that some patients with chronic pain experience the *hit-by-truck effect* after the first one or two triggerband treatments. This transient but dramatic increase in symptoms is a good prognostic sign and is an indication that the injured fascia has been anatomically encountered.

Most injured patients, with the exception of those with tectonic fixations, benefit from the application of ice applied directly to the skin. The preferred method of treatment is a Dixie® cup that has been filled with water and allowed to freeze. The top of the cup is torn away and the skin is massaged with the exposed ice.

Tectonic fixations, unlike the other fascial distortion types, benefit from moist heat. But please note *heat may make every other type of injury worse*. And never apply heat to an acute injury, ever!

ORGANIC DISORDERS

Fascial distortions are thought to occur throughout the body. The coronary arteries, for instance, have both cylinder fascia and fascial bands. It seems reasonable to postulate that if the fascial anatomy of the coronary artery is similar to that of other parts of the body, then the same structural pathological processes found elsewhere would also affect coronary arteries. Perhaps in the future, heart attacks and asthma, renal colic and hypertension, osteoarthritis and osteoporosis, and countless other medical conditions will be envisioned and treated as pathological processes secondary to fascial distortions.

SECTION TWO

TREATMENT OF SPECIFIC CONDITIONS

Chapter 10

THE ORTHOPATHIC TREATMENT OF CERVICAL, THORACIC, AND LUMBAR STRAINS

CERVICAL STRAINS

The most common neck complaints with their associated fascial distortions include:

Complaint	Distortion
Pulling pain from mid-upper back to neck	Star triggerband
Pulling pain from shoulder to neck	Upper trapezius triggerband
Deep ache in supraclavicular fossa	SCHTP
Spot(s) of pain	Continuum distortion
Ache deep in spine	Folding distortion
Spasms or generalized discomfort	Cylinder distortion
Stiffness and tightness of joints	Facet tectonic fixation

Triggerband Cervical Strains

"Pulling" or "burning" pain in the neck is a strong indication that a triggerband is present. The two most frequently encountered neck triggerbands are the *star* and the *upper trapezius* (also known as the *shoulder to mastoid*) triggerbands.

The star triggerband is the most common triggerband found in the human body and particularly in women, is frequently a culprit in neck aches, upper back pain, and sore shoulders. Its symptoms of pain deep under the occiput with a burning or pulling pain from the upper back to the neck is directly attributable to its pathway. It begins halfway between the medial border of the scapula and the thoracic spine at the T6 level and ends either at the ipsilateral mastoid (most fibers) or contralateral mastoid (some fibers).

Triggerband technique of the star can be performed with the patient either sitting or prone. The treatment itself consists of using the physician's thumb to iron out the wrinkled fascial fibers along the entire triggerband pathway from the starting point to the mastoid. The vector of force from the thumb is initially deep into the tissue, but once the triggerband is coaxed to *move* the force becomes both anterior and superior. Note that *movement* of the triggerband means that the twist of the separated fibers is changing locations along the pathway as the fibers are physically re-approximated (re-zipping the Ziploc® bag).

As the treatment continues, the distorted fascial band is palpably followed along its pathway upward to the base of the neck and then to either the ipsilateral or contralateral mastoid. If you are unsure if you are on the pathway, ask the patient, "Am I still on it?" Most people will give a clear and unambiguous answer that will help guide the treatment. At the base of the occiput, the fascial fibers dive deep below the edge of the skull. To follow the triggerband through this area, be sure that your thumb applies strong and deep pressure.

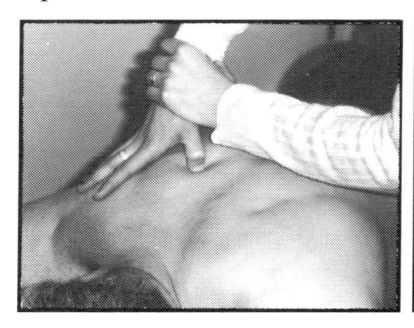

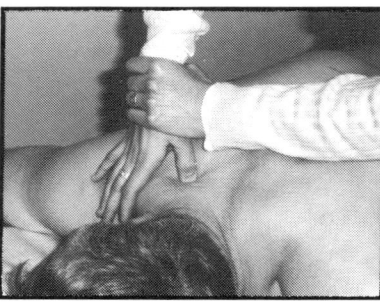

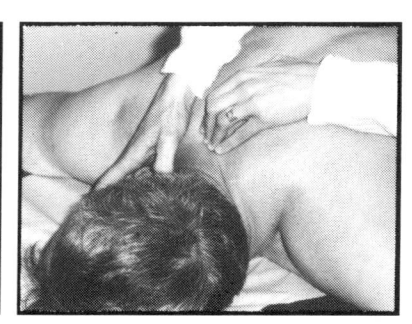

Figure 10-1. Treatment of Star Triggerband

The upper trapezius triggerband is responsible for the burning or pulling sensation from the tip of the shoulder to the mastoid on the same side. It is treated with triggerband technique along its entire pathway with particularly strong force employed along the margin of the superior lateral neck.

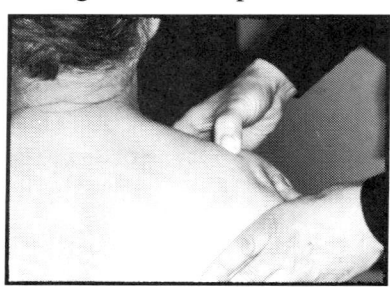

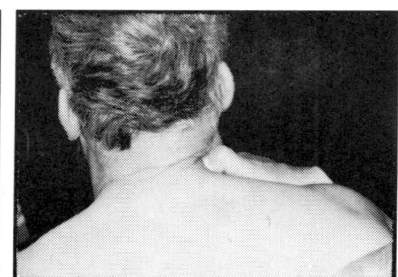

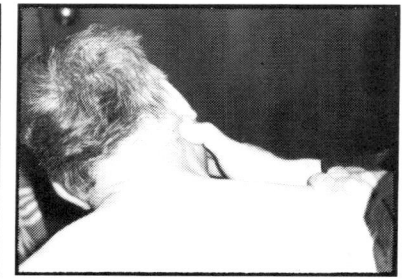

Figure 10-2. Treatment of Upper Trapezius (Shoulder to Mastoid) Triggerband

SCHTP Cervical Strains

Neck aches in which the head is tilted to the side of pain are often the result of the supraclavicular herniated triggerpoint (SCHTP). Note that the SCHTP has two main presentations:

1. In an SCHTP sore shoulder there is typically an associated loss of shoulder internal rotation or abduction
2. In an SCHTP neck ache the clinical finding is altered cervical rotation

The treatment of the SCHTP is discussed in Chapter 4. Note that the goal of the technique is to have the treating thumb apply sufficient pressure directly into the supraclavicular fossa to push the protruding tissue below the fascial plane.

Continuum Cervical Strains

Continuum distortions in the neck generally hurt at the origin and insertion of the cervical ligaments. The most common cause of continuum cervical strain is an auto accident in which there is a jolt to the neck and the ligaments connecting the vertebral transverse processes become injured. Some accidents result in continuum distortions at each vertebral level, which upon palpation seem to line up like a *stack of coins*.

Continuum technique in the neck is best done in the seated position. The doctor stands to the side and palpates the cervical spine with one hand and uses the other hand for the forehead to rest on. The palpating hand cradles the neck so that the thumb is on one side and the fingers on the other. The cervical vertebrae are rocked back and forth between the physician's thumb and middle finger until the continuum distortion is isolated. Then the thumb-tip is focused into the distortion and substantial pressure is held until the release occurs (the transition zone shifts).

In a whiplash injury, inverted distortions are more common than everted distortions, but either is possible. As discussed in Chapter 5, treated inverted distortions may seem to spontaneously regenerate hours later when the transition zone shifts again and the symptoms redevelop. This reoccurrence can often be prevented by delivering high-velocity low-amplitude osteopathic manipulation (HVLA) directly into the treated inverted continuum distortion. However, please note that everted distortions are made worse by HVLA, so if you are unable to distinguish between the two, initially treat only with continuum technique. If the next day there is still pain, treat again with continuum technique followed by HVLA. If instead the neck feels tight or the joints feel stiff (these symptoms signify a concurrent facet tectonic fixation), treat only with HVLA (neutral thrust).

Folding Cervical Strains

Accidents that cause the cervical spine to unfold and torque result in unfolding distortions. The mechanism of injury is often a motor vehicle accident in which the head is thrown forward when the car is struck from behind. The shoulder harness holds the thorax with the trunk slightly flexed as the neck is propelled in the direction of the windshield. The fascia unfolds (and rotates because the force is practically never perfectly centered, nor is the head) and then snaps back into the refolded position contorted.

Refolding distortions occur in a similar manner. The difference is that the neck is restricted from unfolding so the cervical spine is compressed instead of elongated. This injury occurs frequently in car accidents in which the shoulder harness is either loose or absent and the head strikes the windshield. The main symptom of cervical folding injuries is aching deep in the spine. Treatment of unfolding injuries involves traction of the neck, while refolding injuries are corrected with compression. In either case, folding technique is accompanied with HVLA manipulation (see Chapter 6).

Cylinder Cervical Strains

Neck spasms are a sure sign of cylinder distortions and are best treated with double thumb cylinder technique directly over the symptomatic area. Treatment sequence of each layer consists of three steps:
1. Thumbs are placed side-by-side and 1/2 to 1 inch apart
2. Traction is maintained on the skin to pull the cylinder coils apart
3. Release is felt (coils untangle)

Treat the deep layer first by positioning the thumbs medial and lateral to the spasm. Traction and hold until the release, then treat the superficial layer. This is done in the same manner except that the thumbs are positioned above and below the spasm. Remember that the release of a cylinder distortion is small and the palpatory sensation subtle. If the results are less than anticipated, change the treatment to double thumb compression cylinder variant.

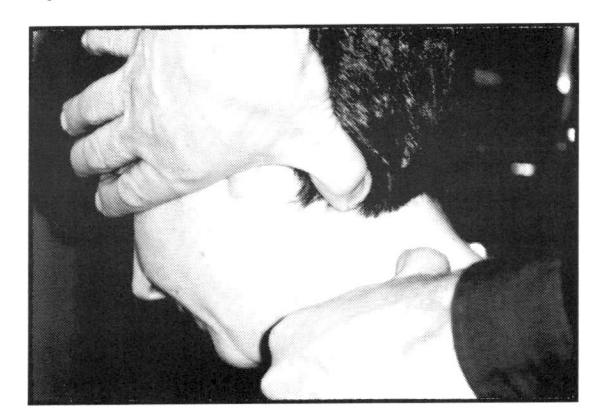

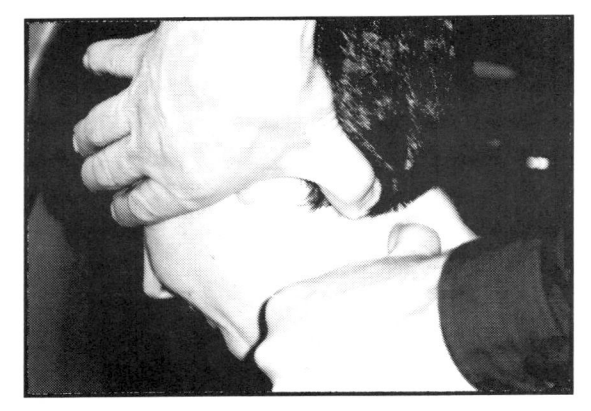

Figure 10-3. Double Thumb Compression Cylinder Variant

If the description of the discomfort is vague, diffuse, difficult to locate, bizarre, or jumps from one area to another, this also indicates that a cylinder distortion is involved. Treatment for these cylinder symptoms is squeegee technique. Use the palm of your hand and plenty of force to slide along the symptomatic areas.

Tectonic Cervical Strains

Tectonic fixations of the facet joints can be either chronic (i.e., secondary to triggerbands with adhesions) or acute. If the injury is chronic, use triggerband technique to fracture the adhesions and forcibly re-approximate the separated portions of the fascial fibers. Then deliver a neutral thrust (no traction or compression) high-velocity low-amplitude manipulation directly into the fixated facet joint. If the tectonic fixation is acute (i.e., there are no triggerbands with adhesions) then a neutral thrust manipulation is all that is necessary. Be aware that acute facet tectonic fixations occur during whiplash injuries if the surrounding joint fluid is forced aside by the facet joints being rammed together.

THORACIC STRAINS

The most common upper back complaints and associated fascial distortions include:

Complaint	Distortion
Pulling pain from mid-upper back to neck	— Star triggerband
Pulling pain from shoulder to neck	— Upper trapezius triggerband
Pulling pain medial to lateral across upper back	— Posterior shoulder triggerband pathway
Deep ache in supraclavicular fossa	— SCHTP
Spot(s) of pain	— Continuum distortion
Ache deep in spine	— Folding distortion
Aching in mid-upper back just medial to scapula	— Star folding
Tightness between first and second ribs	— First rib refolding distortion
Spasm or generalized discomfort	— Cylinder distortion
Stiffness or tightness of joints	— Facet tectonic fixation

Triggerband Thoracic Strains

There are three triggerbands found commonly in thoracic strain:
1. Star
2. Upper trapezius (shoulder to mastoid)
3. Posterior shoulder pathway

The star and the upper trapezius triggerbands are discussed under the section on cervical strain. Note that some patients with the upper trapezius or star triggerband will have neck pain while others will have thoracic pain. This is because a distorted fascial band can cause symptoms anywhere along its pathway. Regardless of where the symptoms are, the treatment is the same — correct the triggerband along its entire pathway.

The posterior shoulder pathway also can be a cause of thoracic strain. These patients commonly complain of a burning pain across their upper back. The associated body language is a sweeping motion with the hand from the posterior shoulder to the base of the contralateral neck or mastoid. (If the complaint is of a sore shoulder instead of upper back pain, then the body language is a sweeping motion along the posterior shoulder or upper arm.)

The posterior shoulder pathway is corrected by triggerband technique from the starting point (proximal/posterior forearm) superiorly through the lateral upper arm and shoulder, across the back, to the contralateral mastoid. Anatomically, there is individual variance in the thoracic course of this triggerband, so as the fibers traverse the spine they may do so at any level between T1 and T4.

Figure 10-4. Treatment of Posterior Shoulder Triggerband Pathway

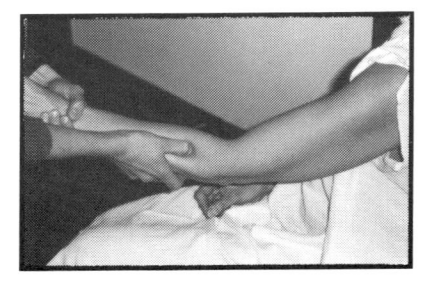

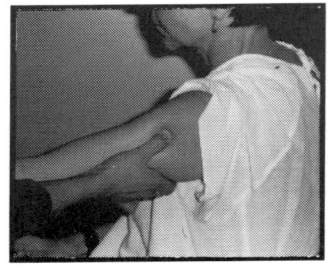

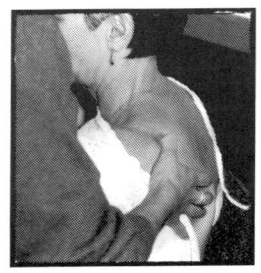

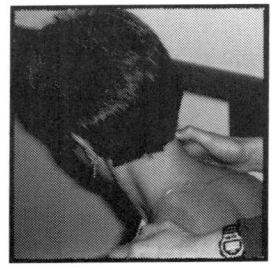

SCHTP Thoracic Strains

The SCHTP can be the culprit in thoracic pain as well as cervical strains and sore shoulders. It is discussed in most detail in Chapter 4. However, if there are concurrent distortions in cervical, thoracic, or shoulder strains, the SCHTP is best treated first.

Continuum Thoracic Strains

Continuum distortions hurt in spots along the transverse processes, the spinous processes, or the ribs. Treatment is with continuum technique, i.e., guiding the vertebra or rib into the position in which the distortion can be most directly palpated, placing the thumb-tip on the distortion, and applying firm pressure until the release (transition zone shifts). Since most of the distortions are inverted, HVLA can be used as an adjunct modality.

Folding Thoracic Strains

In the upper back there are three common folding distortions:
1. Paravertebral
2. Star
3. First rib

Thoracic paravertebral folding distortions occur as a result of accidents similar to those which produce cervical paravertebral folding distortions — that is, from the spine being thrust forward causing the fascia to unfold, torque and refold contorted (unfolding); or the fascia is compressed contorted and can't unfold completely (refolding). Uncorrected folding distortions of the thoracic and lumbar spine are the number one cause of so-called chronic back pain.

Orthopathic treatments (see Chapter 6):
       Upper thoracic unfolding – hallelujah maneuver
       Upper thoracic refolding – chair technique
       Lower thoracic unfolding – wall technique
       Lower thoracic refolding – chair technique

The star folding distortion is located at the star triggerband starting point (intercostal membrane lateral to T6) and should be treated (if present) after the star triggerband is corrected. Since it is an unfolding injury, the manipulative treatment is traction/thrust.

With the patient prone, one treating hand is placed above the superior rib and the other below the inferior rib. Traction is maintained for several seconds followed by a thrust with each hand to unfold the intercostal membrane. If done properly, a pop will be heard as the intercostal membrane unfolds.

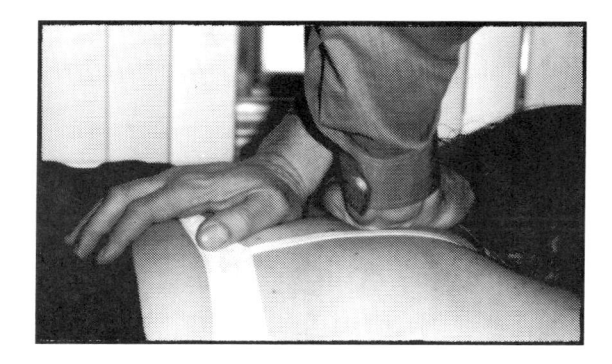

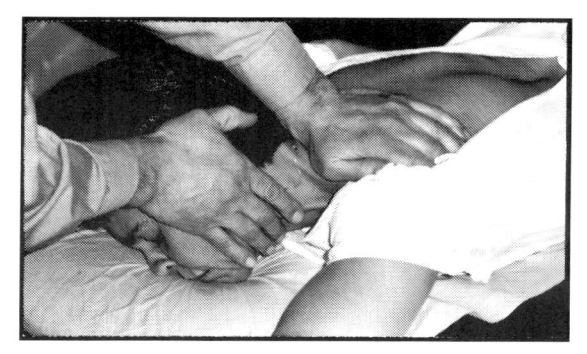

Figure 10-5. Star Unfolding (left) and First-Rib Refolding (right) Manipulations

In the FDM, the first-rib lesion is generally a refolding distortion which causes tightness along the margin of the upper ribs. There are several corrective thrusting modalities to choose from, but ideally each should force the superior rib to push the intercostal membrane together so that it can snap apart as it unfolds. Perhaps the most effective first-rib refolding manipulation is performed with the patient prone and one arm at the side of the body, and the other arm (side of the rib to be treated) abducted (swimmer's position). Compression is applied to the first rib with the palmar aspect of the osteopath's hand (left hand if treating the left first rib) as the other palm cradles the ear. A scissors-like traction is maintained between the rib and neck and then a thrust is made into the rib. When the procedure is successful, a pop (or several pops) will be heard and felt.

Cylinder Thoracic Strains

Just as with cylinder cervical strains, spasm signifies a cylinder distortion. Small areas of spasm can be treated with double thumb cylinder technique. Large or diffuse areas seem to respond better to the squeegee approach. In either case, it is almost always necessary to treat both the left and right sides of the upper back.

Tectonic Thoracic Strains

Two basic facet tectonic fixations occur and identify themselves by direction (horizontal and vertical) based on how they respond to treatment. Horizontal tectonics are treated with the patient positioned either supine or prone (see Figure 8-5):
    Supine - Kirksville crunch (known as *dog technique* in some parts of Europe)
    Prone - Double pisiform thrust

Vertical tectonics are treated standing or sitting with the chair neutral thrust being perhaps the best known example.

Fibromyalgia

In the FDM, when there is a conglomeration of thoracic fascial distortions, this is called fibromyalgia. The physical findings always include triggerbands with adhesions (which make the injury chronic), the SCHTP, and paravertebral folding distortions. However, other fascial distortions are common, including continuum distortions and tectonic fixations. In extreme cases, symptoms of cylinder distortions are so prominent that they confuse the medical diagnosis by adding bizarre objective findings and neurologic-like complaints to the clinical presentation (see Case History #18).

In fibromyalgia there is an initial injury (likely a folding) which goes uncorrected. The loss of the shock-absorbing capability of the paravertebral folding fascia causes surrounding fascial bands to distort when excess forces are exerted upon them. Because they are functionally shorter than when they were uninjured, the newly-formed triggerbands pull other attaching fibers so tightly that those bands (including the fascial fibers around the supraclavicular fossa) also become distorted. Making matters worse, the fractured crosslinks are unable to properly re-align because of the uncorrected and twisted fascial fibers, and eventually heal improperly by attaching to inappropriate structures such as fascial coils, thus causing cylinder distortions. Since the shortened fascial bands pull unevenly on their origins and insertions, continuum distortions develop. And finally, this whole complex of anatomical disarray limits joint movement and allows tectonic fixations to form.

The strategy in treating fibromyalgia is to identify the fascial distortion components and correct them one by one. Triggerbands and the accompanying adhesions as well as the SCHTP should be treated in the first several sessions. Then tectonic fixations and folding distortions are corrected. Once there is sufficient progress with the above, continuum distortions can be addressed. Finally cylinder distortions, if present, are eliminated. Although fibromyalgia is often considered to be incurable and permanent, to the orthopathist each and every case represents a potentially solvable condition.

Low Back Pain

Acute lumbar sprain patients commonly present with one of seven clinical patterns (see Low Back Pain Table). From their complaints and body language each injury can be differentiated into its fascial distortion types and treated with the corresponding fascial distortion techniques.

Triggerbands

If there is a pulling pain down the thigh, a triggerband is strongly suspected and triggerband technique should be initiated along the course of the discomfort. The most common pathway responsible for these symptoms is the *low back pain with thigh tightness triggerband*. It begins 2-3 inches above the knee in the posterior thigh and runs up the middle thigh, over the mid-buttock, past the iliac crest, and onto the low back. Its course then veers medially to the transverse process of L3 or L4 where it loops downward past the sacral base and finally ends at the sacrococcygeal junction.

Low Back Pain Table

Symptom	Body Language	Distortion	Treatment
Pulling pain down back of thigh	Sweeping motion of fingers up and down posterior thigh	Triggerband	Triggerband technique of low back pain with thigh tightness pathway
Pulling pain down lateral thigh	Sweeping motion of fingers up and down iliotibial band	Triggerband	Triggerband technique of lateral thigh triggerband
Pain in buttock	Pushes thumb forcefully into gluteal muscle	Herniated Triggerpoint	Herniated triggerpoint therapy of gluteal bull's-eye
Pain in one spot over SI joint	Points with one finger to PSIS	Inverted Continuum Distortion	Continuum technique followed by thrusting manipulation (scissors technique)
Ache deep in spine	Back of hand is placed against lumbar vertebrae or fist is pushed into lumbar vertebrae	Folding Distortion	Chair technique
Squeezing pain or spasm across low back	Squeezes low back muscles with hands or fingers	Cylinder Distortion	Double thumb cylinder technique
Pain at base of spine	Places hands over iliac crest	Tectonic Fixation	Frogleg and reverse frogleg tectonic techniques

An almost equally common pathway is the *lateral thigh triggerband*. Its starting point is on the lateral thigh one to two inches above the knee. From there it journeys superiorly along the iliotibial tract to the sacroiliac joint. At the SI joint the pathway snakes medially and slightly inferiorly until its fibers reach the sacrum where the pathway terminates.

Herniated Triggerpoint of the Buttocks

The *bull's-eye herniated triggerpoint* is also a cause of what many people call "low back pain." However, when asked to show where they feel the pain, almost all will take a thumb or knuckle and push it into the mid-section of the affected lateral buttock. The bull's-eye HTP is treated with herniated triggerpoint therapy, i.e., the protruding tissue is pushed below the fascial plane by force from the physician's thumb.

However, some patients have the added misfortune of a concurrent everted continuum distortion present just under the HTP. If that is the case, treat the HTP first and then use continuum technique on the continuum distortion. It should be noted that the gluteal continuum distortion is deep below the muscles and against the bone so an extraordinary amount of force is required for correction.

Sacroiliac Joint Continuum Distortions

Another common presentation of "low back pain" is when the patient complains of discomfort in one or several spots over the sacroiliac joint. Since these symptoms signify the presence of inverted continuum distortions, the most successful treatment is continuum technique followed by thrusting manipulation. However, either of these approaches may be quite successful on its own.

Continuum technique is performed with the patient standing, bent at the waist and leaning forward over a counter. The physician pushes his/her thumb-tip directly into the most palpably tender tissue in proximity to the posterior superior iliac spine (PSIS) and holds that force until the distortion releases (i.e., the transition zone shifts).

Thrusting manipulation of the sacroiliac joint can be performed in several different fashions depending on the preference of the treating physician. One particularly effective method has the nickname of the *scissors technique*. For the scissors, the patient is placed on the table in the lateral recumbent position with the head resting on a pillow. When treating the left SI joint, the patient lies on his/her right side with the bottom leg extended and the top hip flexed and knee extended so that the foot drops off the table. The patient's head should be rotated to face the ceiling before thrusting is introduced into the SI joint.

The physician is positioned standing on the side of the table behind the patient and grasps the patient's hand closest to the table with his/her hand. Note that when the left SI joint is to be manipulated the right hand of the physician clasps the right hand of the patient (just like shaking hands). Next, the doctor's other hand is placed over the sacroiliac joint so that the palm abuts against the PSIS.

The correction is made with a firm thrusting force delivered through the palm of the treating hand into the sacroiliac joint. During the thrust, the doctor's non-thrusting hand simultaneously pulls the patient's hand toward the physician. These two concurrent motions, of *pushing* the SI joint and *pulling* the patient's hand, create a scissors-like action. When the treatment is successful a large pop is heard.

Folding Distortions of the Lumbar Spine

Patients who complain of a deep ache in the low back and shove the back of their hand or fist onto the lumbar vertebrae are signaling that there is a folding lumbar strain. Treatment consists of sitting folding technique in which the patient straddles a chair. For unfolding injuries traction/thrust manipulation is performed (see Figure 6-5). Refolding lumbar strains are less common, but can also be treated with the chair technique. The difference — compression is utilized rather than traction. Stubborn injuries may benefit from inversion therapy.

Cylinder Lumbar Strains

Cylinder distortions in the lumbar area present as spasm across the low back and tend to be bilateral. Body language suggestive of a cylinder injury is squeezing of the paravertebral muscles with the fingers of both hands. The double thumb approach is typically the most effective treatment (squeegee is another option). First the deeper layer is corrected by having one thumb traction medially and the other laterally. Then the more superficial layer is treated by traction from the thumbs so that one is pulling superiorly and the other inferiorly. Generally, both the left and right sides are treated with cylinder technique. Treat the most painful side first, and then treat the opposite side. Start with the most superior fascia lateral to L1, then treat lateral to L3, and finally lateral to L5.

In those patients with spasm that doesn't respond to the double thumb traction approach, use the double thumb compression cylinder variant. This treatment is performed in a similar manner except that the two thumbs force the cylinder coils together rather than pull them apart. The compression is held until there is release (small but perceptible lessening in tissue tautness).

Tectonic Fixations of the Hip

Long-standing "low back pain" which presents as a deep ache at the base of the spine is commonly caused by a tectonic fixation of the hip. The body language of wrapping the hands around the iliac crest with the thumbs touching the sacroiliac joint is typical. Treatment consists of first correcting any other distortions (particularly triggerbands) and then performing frogleg and reverse frogleg manipulations (see Figure 8-4).

Body Language and Treatments

	Triggerband	Triggerband	Herniated Triggerpoint
Body Language	Sweeping motion of fingers up and down posterior thigh	Sweeping motion of fingers up and down lateral thigh	Pushes thumb or fingers forcefully into gluteal muscle
Treatments	Triggerband technique of the low back pain with thigh tightness pathway	Triggerband technique of lateral thigh triggerband (a.k.a. iliotibial pathway)	Herniated triggerpoint therapy of gluteal bull's-eye

For Low Back Pain

Continuum Distortion	Folding Distortion	Cylinder Distortion	Tectonic Fixation
Points with one finger to SI joint	Fist or back of hand pushes into lumbar vertebrae	Squeezes low back muscles	Places hands over iliac crests
Continuum technique	Chair technique	Double thumb cylinder technique of deep cylinder fascia	Frogleg tectonic technique
Scissors technique		Double thumb cylinder technique of superficial cylinder fascia	Reverse frogleg tectonic technique

CHRONIC LOW BACK PAIN

As is the case with other types of chronic pain, the treatment of non-organic chronic low back pain (LBP) begins by first fracturing fascial adhesions (to make the injury acute) and then correcting the acute injury. Therefore on every chronic LBP patient the first one or two treatment sessions should include triggerband technique. Treatment with the comb also should be considered. Once the fascial adhesions have been either greatly reduced or eliminated, the patient is re-evaluated and the back injury is broken down into its fascial distortion components and treated with the associated FDM techniques. Note once again that many cases of so-called chronic low back pain (and chronic upper back pain) are anatomically the result of long-standing uncorrected acute folding distortions (no adhesions).

Chapter 11

THE ORTHOPATHIC TREATMENT OF THE SORE SHOULDER

Although wading through the myriad of sore shoulder complaints may seem confounding, each particular injury can be broken down into its fascial distortion components and treated with fascial distortion techniques. For this reason, it is anticipated that virtually every sore shoulder, from acutely sprained to chronically frozen, will make good progress when orthopathically treated.

In contrast to the orthopedic approach which focuses on entrapment, swelling, and tears (i.e., impingement, inflammation, and rotator cuff injuries), the orthopathic approach views the injured shoulder as being the result of one or more fascial distortions which can be manually corrected. This difference in perspective can be illustrated by looking at a specific example, such as a sore shoulder in which the pain is along the bicipital groove. The traditional diagnosis would likely be bicipital tendonitis (i.e., inflammation of the bicipital tendon), whereas the orthopathic diagnosis is *triggerband sore shoulder*.

The terminology chosen in describing this condition (and all sore shoulders) is more than just an issue of semantics — it ultimately influences our treatment choices. For instance, in the example of bicipital groove shoulder pain, the diagnosis of tendonitis typically leads to a cascade of treatment options to fight inflammation (anti-inflammatory medicines, resting, steroid injections, etc.). In contrast, the diagnosis of triggerbands leads to treating with triggerband technique.

SORE SHOULDER BODY LANGUAGE

In order to select the appropriate clinical approach, the orthopathist must be able to differentiate (and appreciate) each of the six principal fascial distortion types that commonly cause sore shoulders. Although subjective complaints, mechanisms of injury, and objective findings are also utilized in the diagnostic process, the initial impression of body language is perhaps the most reliable single indicator of the underlying fascial pathology. In the sore shoulder there are eleven typical presentations, which with practice can be instantly recognized (see Figure 11-1).

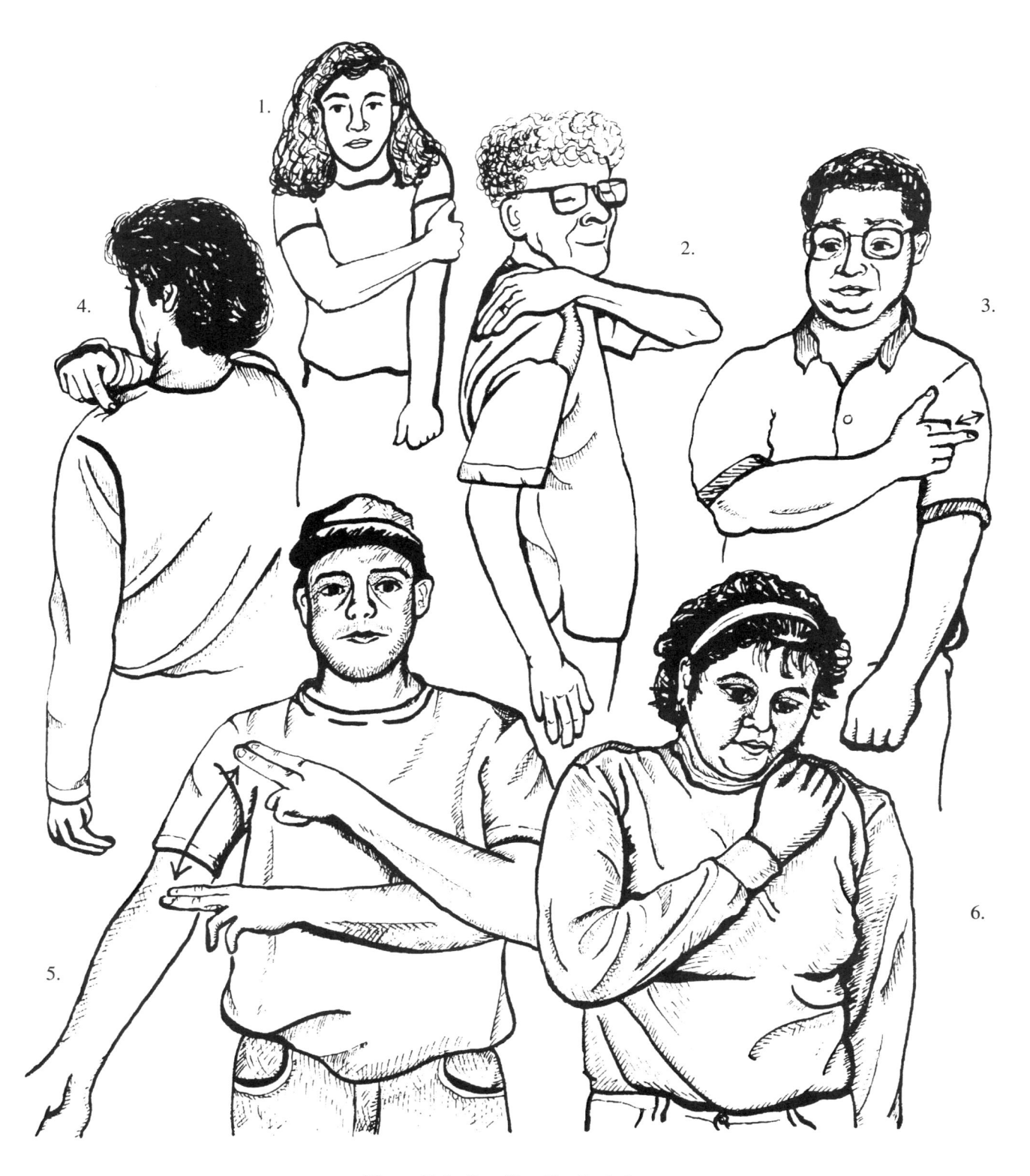

Figure 11-1. Sore Shoulder Body Language

Eleven sore shoulder body language signals: 1. Squeezes upper arm (cylinder distortion), 2. Sweeping motion with fingers from mid-back to mastoid (star triggerband), 3. Rubs finger laterally across humeral neck (refolding distortion), 4. Pointing to spot of pain with one finger (continuum distortion), 5. Sweeping motion with fingers along anterior shoulder (anterior shoulder triggerband pathway), 6. Fingers pressing into the supraclavicular fossa (SCHTP).

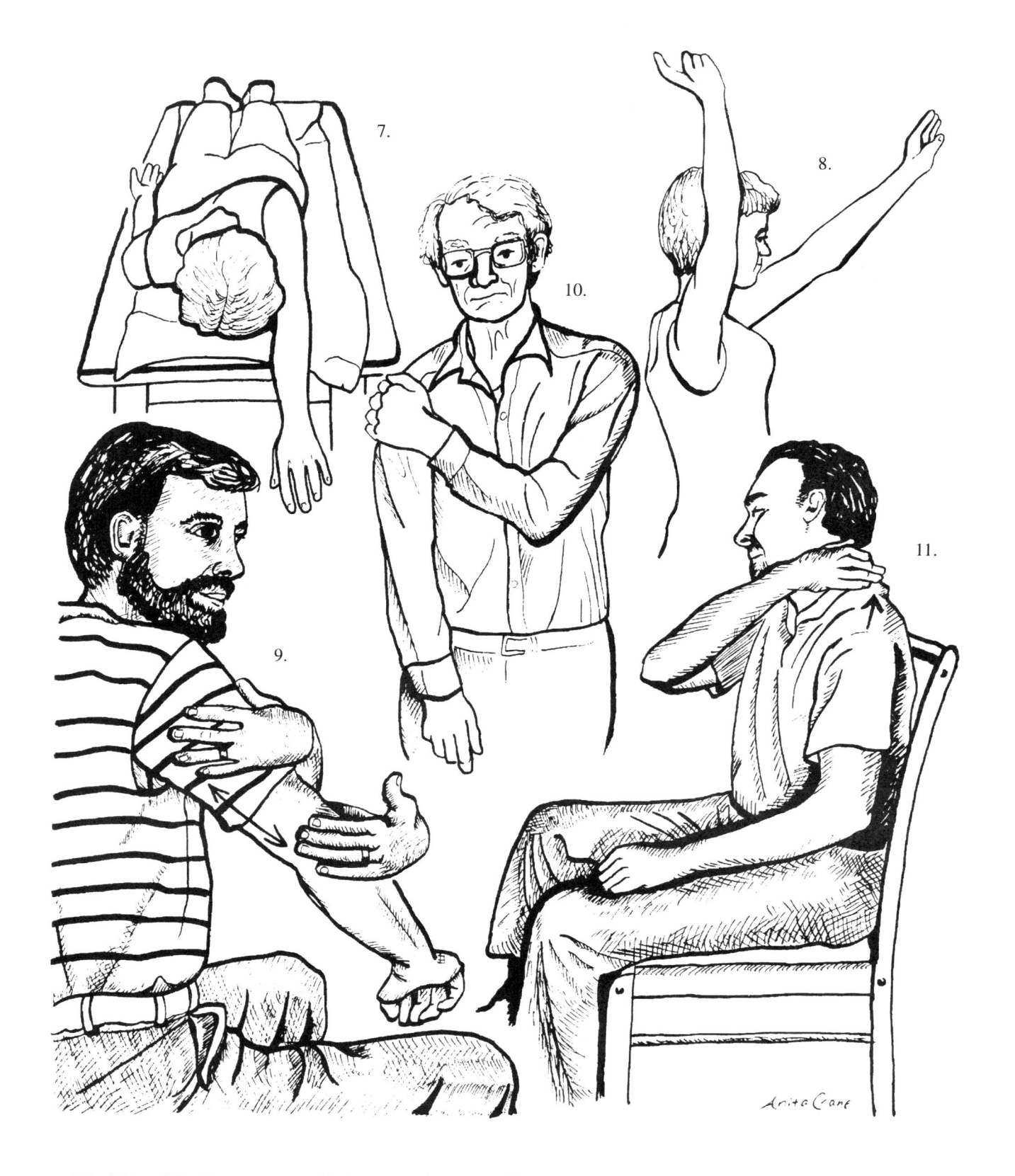

7. Inability of shoulder to contact table in prone swimmers position (tectonic fixation), 8. Inability to abduct shoulder without concurrent forward flexion (tectonic fixation), 9. Sweeping motion with hand along posterior shoulder (posterior shoulder triggerband pathway), 10. Squeezes shoulder joint (unfolding or refolding distortion), 11. Sweeping motion with fingers from shoulder to mastoid (upper trapezius triggerband).

VERBAL DESCRIPTIONS OF SHOULDER PAIN

Despite the apparent complexity of verbal shoulder complaints, there are key words and descriptions which patients make that can be correlated to the specific underlying fascial distortions.

Triggerbands	—	Pulling or burning pain on front of arm (anterior shoulder pathway)
	—	Pulling or burning pain down back of arm (posterior shoulder pathway)
	—	Pulling or burning pain from shoulder to mastoid (upper trapezius triggerband)
	—	Pulling or burning pain from upper back to neck (star triggerband)
Herniated Triggerpoints (SCHTP)	—	Achy-tightness over shoulder
Continuum Distortions	—	Spot(s) of pain
Folding Distortions	—	Aching deep in joint
Cylinder Distortions	—	Pain (tightness, spasm, or ache) in upper arm
Tectonic Fixations	—	Stiffness in shoulder, shoulder joint is "dry" or "needs to be lubricated"

EVALUATING MOTION OF THE SORE SHOULDER

In the shoulder, all six principal fascial distortion types are possible. In order to be able to understand their presentations so that they can be adequately differentiated and treated, it is advisable to know which motions each distortion type might affect. Fortunately, there are typically only three shoulder motions which are clinically relevant. These are abduction, external rotation, and internal rotation.

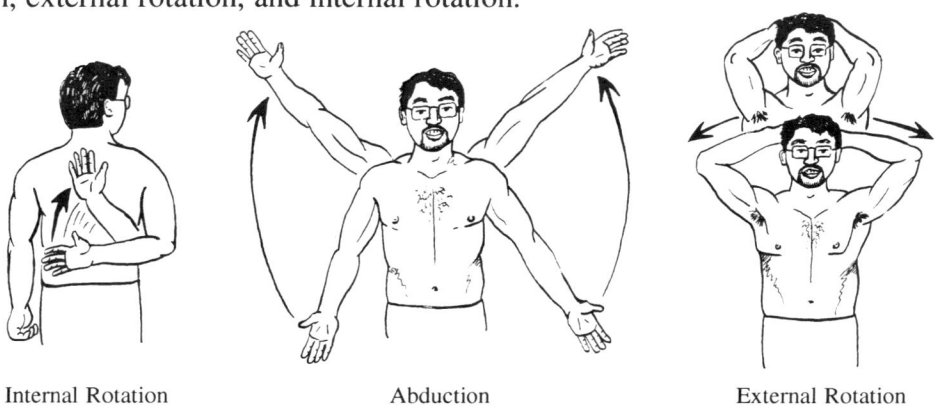

Internal Rotation   Abduction   External Rotation
Figure 11-2. Three Important Shoulder Motions

Abduction is the motion in which the hands are brought from the sides of the body up and over the head with the elbows extended. Note that the hands are allowed to rotate so that the palms begin flat against the thighs and end flat against each other above the head. External rotation is the motion that places the elbows posteriorly at the level of the neck. The fingers of each hand are intertwined and the elbows are pushed backwards. Clinically, internal rotation is the most sensitive of all the shoulder motions and is considered to be the ability to place the back of the hand against the back of the body. Loss of internal rotation is the most common physical sign of a sore shoulder (and the most overlooked).

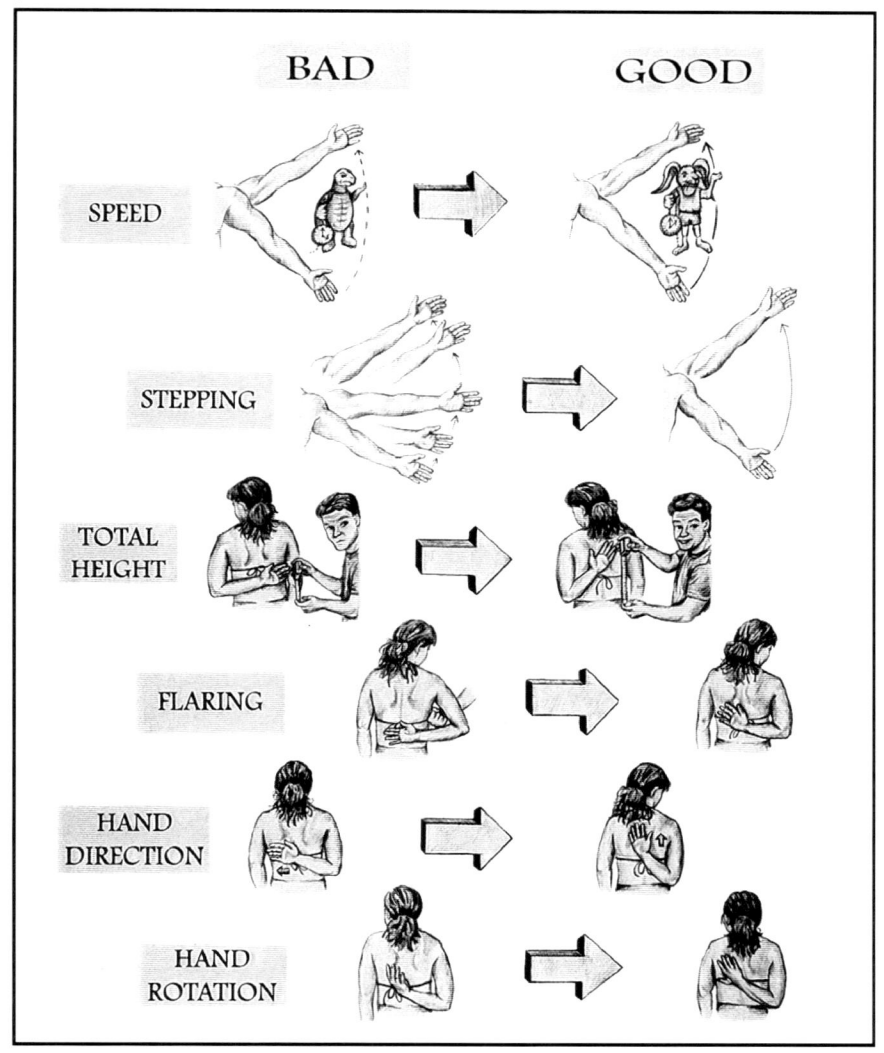

Figure 11-3. Subtle Shoulder Motions

In addition to gross loss of abduction, external, and internal rotation, there are subtle signs of motion which indicate that a fascial distortion is present and that the shoulder is injured. Look for:
- Speed – amount of time it takes to abduct or internally or externally rotate
- Stepping – small jerking motions seen with movement
- Total height – distance above pant line that fingers can reach during internal rotation (measure with a ruler and record number of inches or centimeters)
- Flaring – space between elbow and body present with sub-optimal internal rotation (record number of fingers or fist that can fit through the hole)
- Hand direction – optimal internal rotation includes fingers pointing straight up toward ceiling
- Hand rotation – ability to place the palm of the hand flat against the back of the body

Orthopathic Flow Chart of the Acutely Sore Shoulder

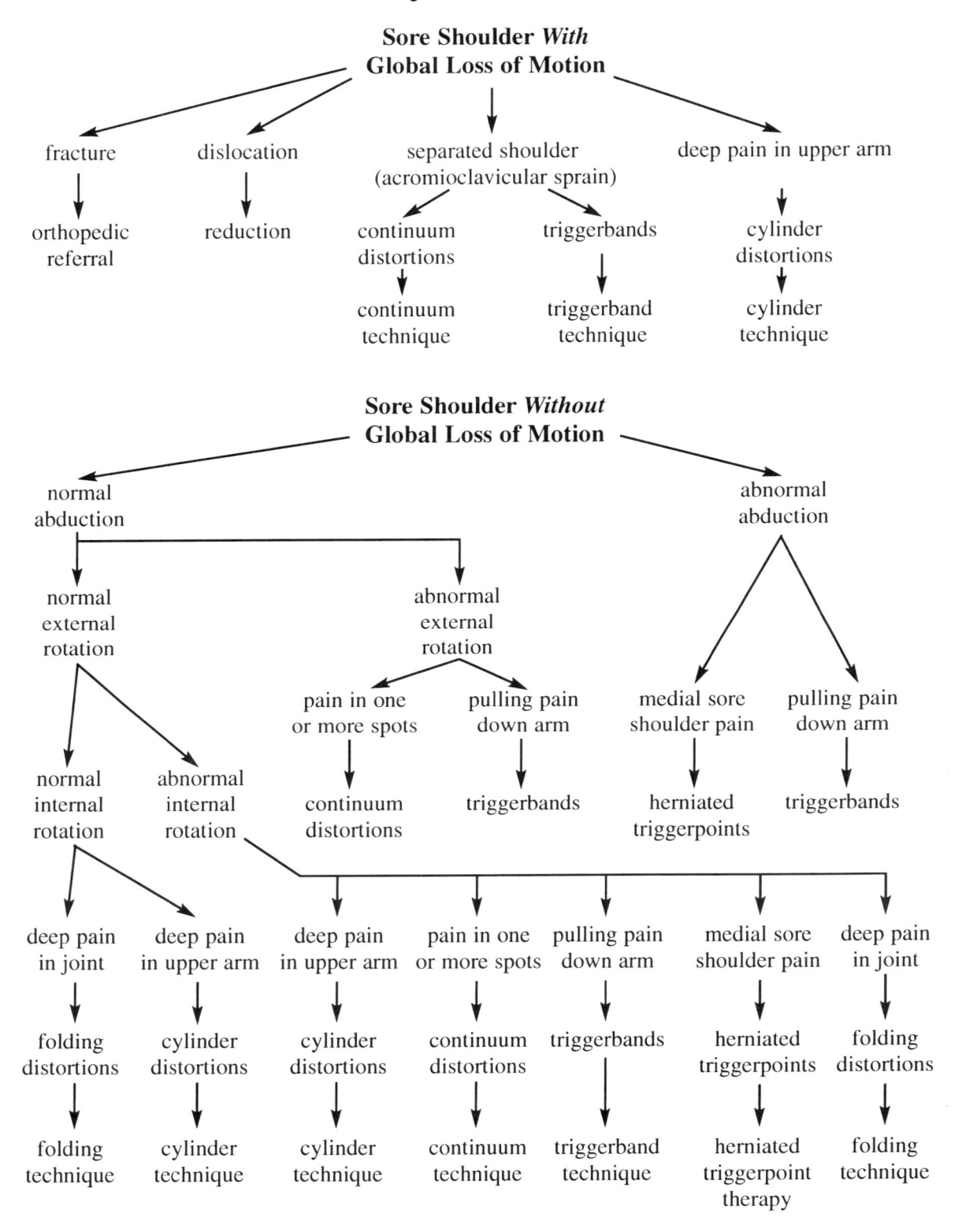

Sore Shoulder *With* Global Loss of Motion

- fracture → orthopedic referral
- dislocation → reduction
- separated shoulder (acromioclavicular sprain)
  - continuum distortions → continuum technique
  - triggerbands → triggerband technique
- deep pain in upper arm → cylinder distortions → cylinder technique

Sore Shoulder *Without* Global Loss of Motion

- normal abduction
  - normal external rotation
    - normal internal rotation
      - deep pain in joint → folding distortions → folding technique
      - deep pain in upper arm → cylinder distortions → cylinder technique
    - abnormal internal rotation
      - deep pain in upper arm → cylinder distortions → cylinder technique
  - abnormal external rotation
    - pain in one or more spots → continuum distortions
    - pulling pain down arm → triggerbands
- abnormal abduction
  - medial sore shoulder pain → herniated triggerpoints
  - pulling pain down arm → triggerbands

Subsequent techniques:
- pain in one or more spots → continuum distortions → continuum technique
- pulling pain down arm → triggerbands → triggerband technique
- medial sore shoulder pain → herniated triggerpoints → herniated triggerpoint therapy
- deep pain in joint → folding distortions → folding technique

Orthopathic Flow Chart of the Chronically Sore Shoulder

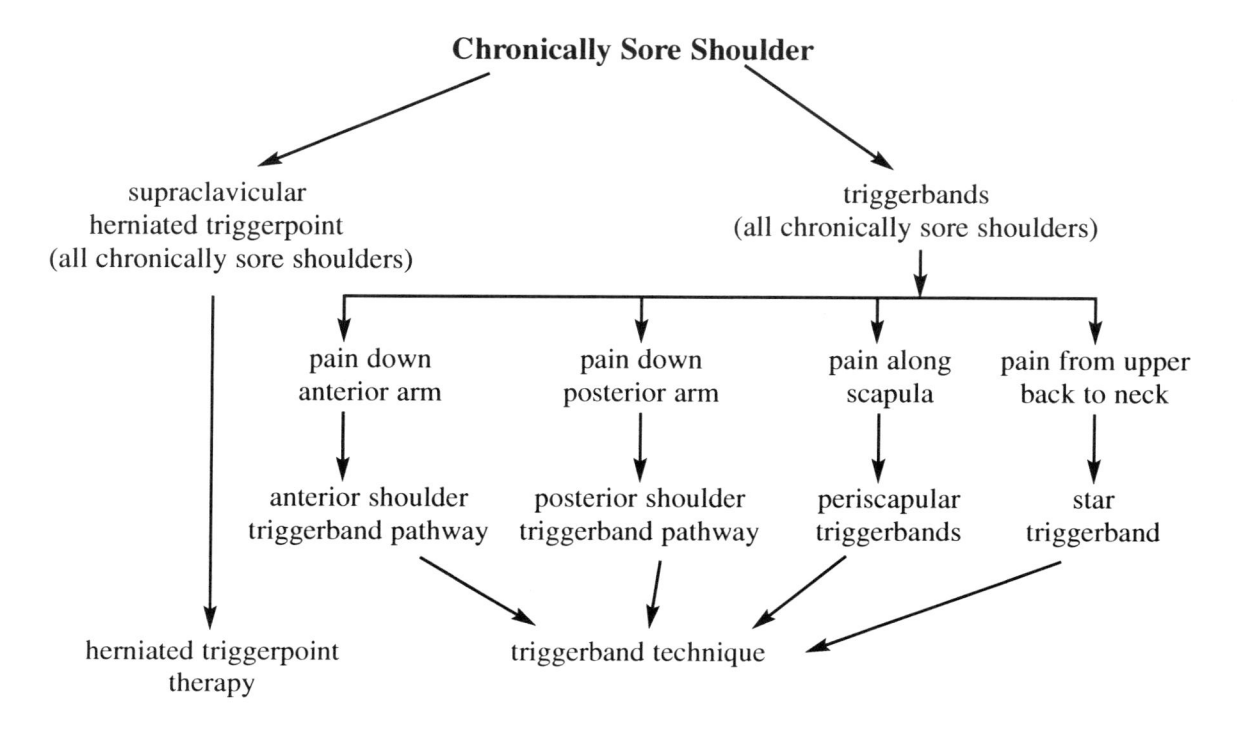

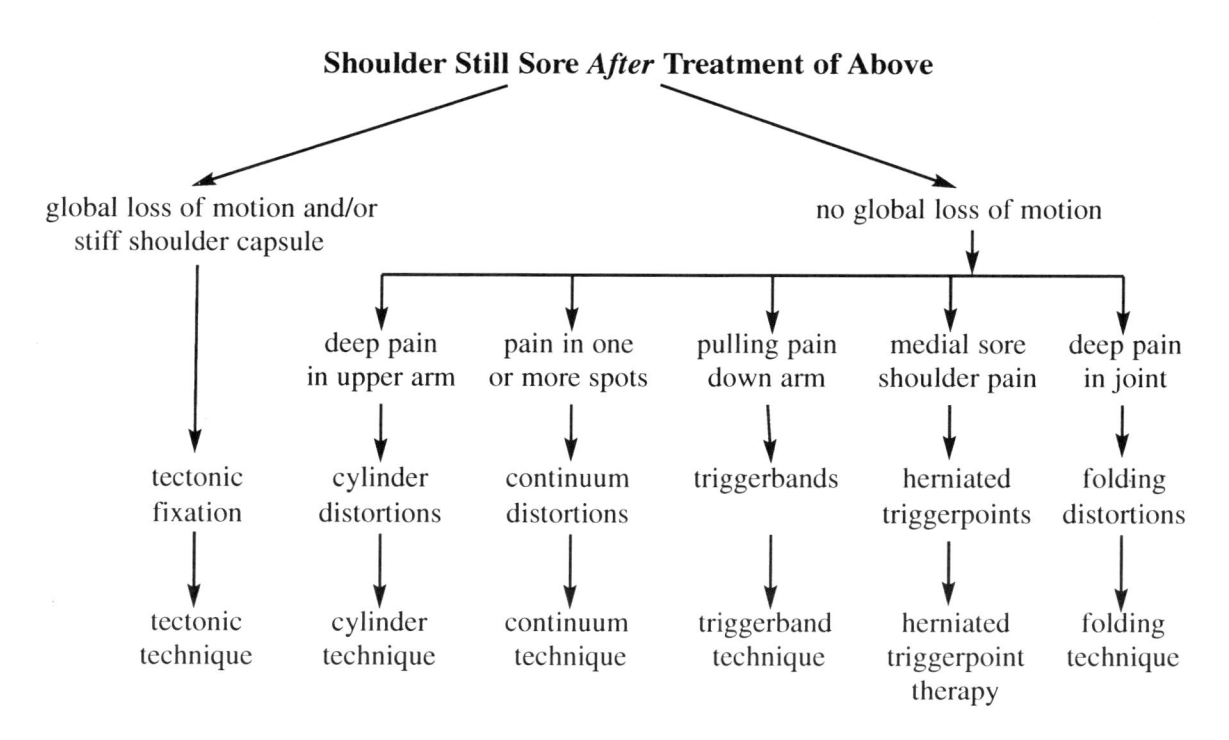

Chronically Sore Shoulder

- supraclavicular herniated triggerpoint (all chronically sore shoulders)
  - → herniated triggerpoint therapy
- triggerbands (all chronically sore shoulders)
  - pain down anterior arm → anterior shoulder triggerband pathway
  - pain down posterior arm → posterior shoulder triggerband pathway
  - pain along scapula → periscapular triggerbands
  - pain from upper back to neck → star triggerband
  - → triggerband technique

Shoulder Still *After* Treatment of Above

- global loss of motion and/or stiff shoulder capsule
  - tectonic fixation → tectonic technique
- no global loss of motion
  - deep pain in upper arm → cylinder distortions → cylinder technique
  - pain in one or more spots → continuum distortions → continuum technique
  - pulling pain down arm → triggerbands → triggerband technique
  - medial sore shoulder pain → herniated triggerpoints → herniated triggerpoint therapy
  - deep pain in joint → folding distortions → folding technique

Loss of shoulder motion, whether it is grossly visible (such as inability to raise the arm) or subtle (such as sluggishness of hand rotation during internal rotation) are physical signs of shoulder dysfunction. Each particular distortion type generally affects shoulder motion in specific ways that can be measured and evaluated. The preceding flow chart matches the fascial distortions with their typical clinical presentations. Please note that any of the distortions can cause loss of internal rotation.

ACUTELY SORE SHOULDERS

Acutely sore shoulders can be clinically divided into two groups: those with global loss of motion (i.e., impairment in all three primary shoulder motions – abduction, external rotation, and internal rotation), and those without global loss of motion. See Orthopathic Flow Chart of the Acutely Sore Shoulder.

Acutely sore shoulders with global loss of motion generally have four etiologies:
1. Fracture
2. Dislocation
3. Separated shoulder (subluxation or dislocation of acromioclavicular joint)
4. Upper arm cylinder distortion

ACUTELY SORE SHOULDERS WITH GLOBAL LOSS OF MOTION

Fractures (Humerus)

Fractures of the shoulder are most likely to be humeral head or neck and are most common in post-menopausal women. These individuals initially present with a sudden onset of substantial pain in the upper arm following a specific incident such as a fall. The typical orthopedic treatment for closed and non-serious fractures is symptomatic (ice and pain medications) with immobilization (sling). The expected outcome of this approach is a gradual diminishing of pain over several months. The orthopedic orthopathist, in contrast, supplements the medical regimen with FDM techniques which are meant to immediately diminish pain, decrease healing time, and allow for earlier mobilization (which lessens the opportunity for tectonic fixations to form). The typical sequence of corrections is:

1. SCHTP (if present)
2. Upper trapezius triggerband (if present)
3. Folding distortions (always present)
4. Continuum distortions (always present)
5. Cylinder distortions (commonly present)

The SCHTP does not occur with every fracture, but if it is present it should be corrected with the patient sitting, not lying. The reason for this is that these patients are unable to tolerate the supine position. Triggerbands, like the SCHTP are only minor components of the total fracture/fascial distortion complex, but also should be treated (if they exist).

The two major fascial distortion components of every humeral fracture are folding and continuum distortions. Folding distortions should be addressed before continuum distortions and occur in two radiological varieties:
1. Those with separated fractured segments
2. Those with compression fractures

The orthopathic treatment approach is gentle unfolding for those with separated segments, and gentle refolding for those with osseous compression. In either case, the procedure requires little brawn, much finesse, and no thrust. Continuum distortions are found in every fracture along the fracture site itself, so continuum technique should be considered for appropriate patients and applied to the most exquisitely tender spots of pain. However, the physician should be aware that this particular procedure is painful, poorly tolerated by patients, and runs the risk of inducing vasovagal responses.

Cylinder distortions are yet another complicating factor in humeral fractures, but fortunately are not found in every case. Treatment consists of either double thumb cylinder technique or double thumb compression cylinder variant (CCV).

Fractures (Clavicular)

Broken collar bones can also cause acute global loss of motion. The typical treatment sequence includes correcting the SCHTP followed by continuum technique of the fracture sites (providing there is no open wound, vascular or nerve impairment, or risk of pneumothorax).

Dislocations (Gleno-humeral)

Dislocations of the gleno-humeral joint are a common condition seen in the Emergency Department. The orthopedic approach is traction (i.e., unfolding technique). Adding finesse to the brawn of this therapy means consciously directing the contorted fascia through the process (i.e., unfolding the fascia and allowing it to pull the head of the humerus back into the glenoid fossa) followed by guided refolding (controlled cessation of traction). Envisioning the correction in this manner often results in a relatively smooth reduction that requires little or no pharmaceutical support.

Separated Shoulders (Acromioclavicular Sprains)

Subluxations and/or dislocations of the acromioclavicular joint clinically present with triggerbands and/or continuum distortions. The body language of triggerband separated shoulders is a sweeping motion of the fingers along portions of the lateral clavicle. In contrast, the body language of continuum distortions consists of pointing with one finger to the spots of pain. Triggerband separated shoulders are obviously treated with triggerband technique (follow the triggerband along the clavicle and correct it over its entire pathway), whereas continuum distortions are treated with continuum technique (apply precise pressure to the small spots of tenderness and hold until the osseous portion of the transition zone shifts). Separated shoulders generally respond well to FDM techniques and the expected result is an immediate reduction in pain and normalization of motion.

Three clinical considerations:
1. Triggerbands and continuum distortions commonly occur in the same injury
2. Ice is an adjunct therapy
3. Re-treatment should be performed the following day to correct residual distortions

Cylinder Distortions (Upper Arm Sprains)

Surprisingly, upper arm cylinder distortions (see Figure 7-1) that cause global loss of motion are perhaps the most painful of all the shoulder injuries (including fractures). Clinically they mimic fractures in the severity of pain and the extent of loss of motion, but can be distinguished from them by a negative x-ray, and history of insidious onset (as opposed to a specific incident which is characteristic of fractures). And in those patients that have retained at least some abduction, cylinder distortions are notorious for eliciting biting pain during adduction.

Cylinder shoulder sprains (also known as cylinder acutely frozen shoulders and cylinder upper arm sprains) are treated in the following manner:

1. Ice massage (with real ice applied directly to the skin) – this is especially critical for those patients who unwisely applied a heating pad or warm wash cloth to the arm or shoulder prior to being seen
2. Double thumb cylinder technique
3. Narcotic pain medicines (appropriate patients only)
4. Ice massage at home every several hours (No heat!)
5. Recheck the next day. Re-treat with double thumb cylinder technique (consider compression cylinder variant and squeegee technique – do not use Indian burn)

Although to the patient the primary concern of a cylinder distortion is pain, he/she should be made aware that self-imposed immobility leads to stiffness (i.e., formation of tectonic fixations).

ACUTELY SORE SHOULDERS WITHOUT GLOBAL LOSS OF MOTION

This group of sore shoulders has two distinct histories: those that had global loss of motion and are being treated, and those that never had global loss of motion. In either case, the orthopathic approach is the same:
- Synthesize the body language, description of pain, mechanism of injury, and physical findings to make an orthopathic diagnosis
- Correct the corresponding fascial distortions

Impaired Abduction in the Acutely Sore Shoulder

The supraclavicular herniated triggerpoint (SCHTP) and the anterior and posterior shoulder triggerband pathways are far and away the most likely culprits responsible for loss of abduction. Fortunately, these patients often have an immediate and impressive response to an aggressive treatment of herniated triggerpoint therapy and/or triggerband technique. Clinically, this rapid and often complete restoration of motion and strength (as well as reduction or elimination of pain) is possible (and expected) even in patients with MRI suggested rotator cuff tears.

Considering the body language and verbal description of discomfort, if the patient complains of tightness or achiness in the supraclavicular fossa (particularly if it is accompanied with the body language of pushing the fingers into the supraclavicular fossa), treat the SCHTP. If instead there is a pulling pain down the anterior arm, with the associated sweeping motion of the fingers along the bicipital groove — treat the anterior shoulder pathway. Or if the pulling pain is down the back of the arm and includes a sweeping motion of the fingers along that course — treat the posterior pathway.

If the exact distortion responsible for loss of abduction is uncertain, treat in this order (recheck abduction after each step):
1. SCHTP
2. Anterior shoulder pathway
3. Posterior shoulder pathway

If abduction is not completely restored, repeat the sequence with extra force. Note that the anterior pathway begins on the anterior proximal forearm and courses up through the bicipital groove, across the clavicle, and up the neck to the ipsilateral mastoid (see Figure 3-3). The posterior pathway has its starting point on the posterior proximal forearm and hooks around the posterior elbow, up the lateral arm, across the posterior shoulder, over the thoracic spine (T1-T4), and finally up the opposite side of the neck to the contralateral mastoid (see Figure 10-4).

Impaired External Rotation in the Acutely Sore Shoulder

Impairment of external rotation is almost certainly due to the presence of either triggerbands or continuum distortions. If triggerbands are involved, the patient will make a sweeping motion with the fingers along the specified pathway (upper trapezius, and anterior and posterior are most common). If instead continuum distortions are to blame, then the patient will point to the spot(s) of pain with one finger.

Impaired Internal Rotation in the Acutely Sore Shoulder

In general, the measurement of internal rotation is the most objective finding to be made in a sore shoulder. Not only can it be physically quantified with a tape measure, but as the motion objectively improves with the treatment, symptoms correspondingly diminish.

And although any of the principal types of fascial distortions (including tectonic fixations, which in the shoulder are chronic) can cause loss of internal rotation, triggerbands and the SCHTP are the most common culprits (see Orthopathic Flow Chart of the Acutely Sore Shoulder).

Normal Motion — But the Shoulder Hurts

These rare injuries are always acute by definition and never involve triggerbands or adhesions. Instead the fascial etiology is a folding distortion of the shoulder (generally unfolding) or cylinder distortion of the upper arm. The treatment is first with traction/thrust or compression/thrust of the shoulder in multiple directions, and if that is ineffective, follow with double thumb cylinder technique or compression cylinder variant of the upper arm.

Normal Motion — and the Shoulder Doesn't Hurt

In the treatment of sore shoulders there are four possible clinical results:
1. Shoulder hurts and has impaired motion
2. Shoulder hurts but has normal motion
3. Shoulder doesn't hurt but has impaired motion
4. Shoulder doesn't hurt and has normal motion

When the shoulder is asymptomatic and there is normal motion, then that shoulder is considered to be uninjured. Although this category may seem obvious, it is important to remember that this is the condition we wish every sore shoulder to attain. The desired outcome of every orthopathic treatment is therefore a shoulder with normal motion that doesn't hurt.

NON-SHOULDER FASCIAL DISTORTIONS

In addition to correcting the injured shoulder, the orthopath should also consider the effect of the instigating injury on adjacent structures. In particular the following fascial distortions tend to accompany shoulder injuries and should be treated if present:
- Cervical folding distortions
- Cervical facet tectonic fixations
- Upper thoracic folding distortions
- Thoracic facet tectonic fixations
- Star triggerband
- Star folding
- First-rib folding

Treatment of these injuries is generally with high-velocity low-amplitude osteopathic manipulation (with the exception of the star triggerband) and is discussed in chapters 6, 8, and 10.

CHRONICALLY FROZEN SHOULDERS

All chronically frozen or sore shoulders clinically exhibit triggerbands with adhesions and the supraclavicular herniated triggerpoint. Therefore the approach in treating is three-fold:
1. Anatomically eliminate the SCHTP
2. Break adhesions to make the injury acute
3. Correct the remaining distortions

Correction of the SCHTP should be the first objective in treating every chronically frozen shoulder. The next goal is to iron out the affected triggerbands (particularly the star, upper trapezius, and anterior and posterior pathways). Note that the upper trapezius triggerband (and in some cases the posterior pathway) has fibers which traverse the posterior margin of the supraclavicular fossa. The adhesions of these triggerbands *cement* onto the SCHTP and keep it from releasing, while at the same time the SCHTP is distorting the fascial fibers, causing triggerbands. This combination of herniated triggerpoints and triggerbands with adhesions is clinically demonstrated by the need to re-treat the SCHTP and triggerbands over several sessions.

Global Loss of Motion After Treatment of Triggerbands and SCHTP

Once the SCHTP and triggerbands have been corrected (or at least partially eliminated) the motion of the shoulder can be more appropriately evaluated. If the shoulder had global loss of motion before the initiation of the treatment and still does after the SCHTP and triggerbands are corrected, then the primary underlying distortion is a tectonic fixation. Note that these patients have:
1. Stiff shoulders that during abduction exhibit anterior rotation and flexion
2. A fist of space or more between the surface of the table and the shoulder joint when laid prone in the swimmers position (see Figure 11-1)

Sequence of treatment modalities for shoulder tectonic fixations is:
1. Herniated triggerpoint therapy and triggerband technique
2. Slow tectonic pump
3. Frogleg and reverse frogleg tectonic technique
4. Slow tectonic pump
5. Frogleg and reverse frogleg tectonic technique
6. Slow tectonic pump
7. Consider utilizing:
   A. Unfolding or refolding techniques combined with slow tectonic pump
   B. Prone tectonic technique (see glossary term *Prone Tectonic Technique of the Shoulder*)
   C. Plunger technique
   D. Heating of shoulder with hot wet towel prior to frogleg/reverse frogleg techniques

E. Cupping (oriental form of treatment in which suction cups are applied and held onto the shoulder by creating a vacuum with an air extraction gun – see glossary term *Cupping*) combined with other tectonic techniques
F. Whip technique (see Figure 11-9)
G. Brute force tectonic techniques in which the full weight of the physician is directed onto the shoulders or scapula (see Figure 11-9)

Tectonic fixations are generally the most difficult of all the distortions to correct in a chronically frozen shoulder. The primary reason for this is that in addition to the attractive magnetic field suctioning the joint surfaces together, there is the added physical problem of the thickened synovial fluid inhibiting joint sliding.

No Global Loss of Motion — But the Shoulder Still Hurts

Once the SCHTP and triggerbands (and tectonic fixations if they were also present) are corrected, the injury is considered to be acute. The same treatment plan is utilized for these previously chronic sore shoulders as is employed on acutely sore shoulders. Again, the thrust of the process is to determine the residual fascial distortions present and apply the corresponding fascial distortion techniques. Associated regional fascial injuries should also be treated (such as thoracic facet tectonic fixations and first-rib refolding distortions).

GENERAL GUIDELINES IN TREATING THE CHRONICALLY FROZEN SHOULDER

On the average, most chronically sore or frozen shoulders can be corrected with three to seven productive treatment sessions. On each of the first several visits, the SCHTP, the star and upper trapezius triggerbands, and the anterior and posterior pathways should be re-treated. In addition, some frozen shoulders have periscapular triggerbands, continuum distortions, and tectonic fixations which also need to be corrected. The existence of these periscapular distortions (particularly those found along the subscapularis muscle) is suggested by the patient's complaint that the shoulder blade doesn't feel as if it rotates properly.

If a patient with a chronically sore shoulder has multiple complaints and the shoulder itself contains multiple distortions, treat in this order:
1. Herniated triggerpoint therapy
2. Triggerband technique
3. Continuum technique
4. Tectonic technique
5. Folding technique
6. HVLA of regional folding distortions
7. HVLA of regional facet tectonic fixations
8. Cylinder technique

The order in which the three primary shoulder motions return is:
1. Abduction
2. External rotation
3. Internal rotation

Internal rotation generally returns in this order:
1. Total height
2. Hand direction
3. Speed
4. Fluidity
5. Hand rotation

Typical Steps in Treating a Chronically Frozen Sore Shoulder

1. Listen to the history of injury and patient's description of pain.

2. Physical exam – record range of motion including abduction, external rotation, and internal rotation.

3. Diagnostic studies as needed to rule out fracture, multiple myeloma, cancer, or other medical etiologies.

4. Make the diagnosis of chronically frozen shoulder of fascial origin.

5. Consider contraindications to treatment.

6. Discuss the treatment with the patient and explain that it will be painful, bruising may occur, and that he/she can expect to be sore for several days.

7. TREATMENT NUMBER ONE:
    A. SCHTP
    B. Star triggerband
    C. Anterior shoulder pathway (if tightness is in front aspect of shoulder)
    D. Posterior shoulder pathway (if tightness is in posterior aspect of shoulder)
    E. Shoulder to mastoid triggerband (if tightness is along upper trapezius muscle)

8. Allow two to four days before the second treatment. Instruct patient to apply ice and avoid heat.

9. On the second office visit, re-evaluate and record motion.

10. TREATMENT NUMBER TWO:
    A. SCHTP
    B. Star triggerband (if needed)
    C. Anterior shoulder pathway (if needed)

D. Posterior shoulder pathway (if needed)
   E. Continuum distortions if pain in one or more spots
   F. Periscapular triggerbands, continuum distortions, and tectonic fixations (if shoulder blade rotation is abnormal)

11. Several days of rest (usually about three) – use ice and avoid heat.

12. On third office visit, re-evaluate motion and progress.

13. THIRD TREATMENT:
   A. SCHTP (if needed)
   B. Re-treat triggerbands if pulling pain is still present
   C. If the shoulder is still unable to abduct fully, use tectonic technique
   D. If aching deep in joint and there is a history of dislocation or a stretch/pulling injury, use unfolding technique. If aching deep in joint with history of a compression injury, use refolding technique.
   E. Consider high-velocity low-amplitude osteopathic manipulation for regionally associated folding distortions and facet tectonic fixations.
      Cervical spine:
         - Folding distortions – HVLA with concurrent traction or compression (either seated or supine)
         - Tectonic fixations – HVLA with neutral thrust (seated or supine)
      First rib:
         - Refolding distortions – compression/thrust (swimmer's position)
         - Unfolding distortions – modified hallelujah maneuver
      Thoracic spine:
         - Folding distortions – HVLA against wall (unfolding lower thoracic), hallelujah (unfolding upper thoracic), or chair (unfolding or refolding)
         - Tectonic fixations – HVLA (Kirksville crunch or chair neutral thrust)
      Star folding:
         - Unfolding HVLA traction/thrust of intercostal membrane at star triggerband starting point
   F. If motion is normal except internal rotation is slow or hand rotation is poor, consider Indian burn cylinder technique of elbow and forearm.

14. Allow two or three days of rest. Apply ice as needed and avoid heat.

15. Fourth office visit – recheck motion and symptoms.

16. FOURTH TREATMENT:
   Focus attention on remaining distortions. If abduction is slow, re-treat the SCHTP and triggerbands; if hand rotation is limited, then re-treat cylinder distortions; if globally there is little improvement, then treat with tectonic technique; and if pain is deep in joint, use folding technique.

17. Allow a couple days of rest.

18. Fifth office visit. Re-evaluate shoulder motion and progress of treatments.

19. FIFTH TREATMENT:
    A. Treat any motions that are still hesitant
    B. Thrusting manipulation if indicated
    C. If upper arm pain is still present, treat with cylinder technique
    D. Demonstrate to patient objective improvement. To illustrate this point, it may be worthwhile to read the first note from the chart and compare the motion on first exam to current motion.

20. Re-treat as needed.

Figure 11-4. Common Shoulder Triggerband Pathways and Treatments

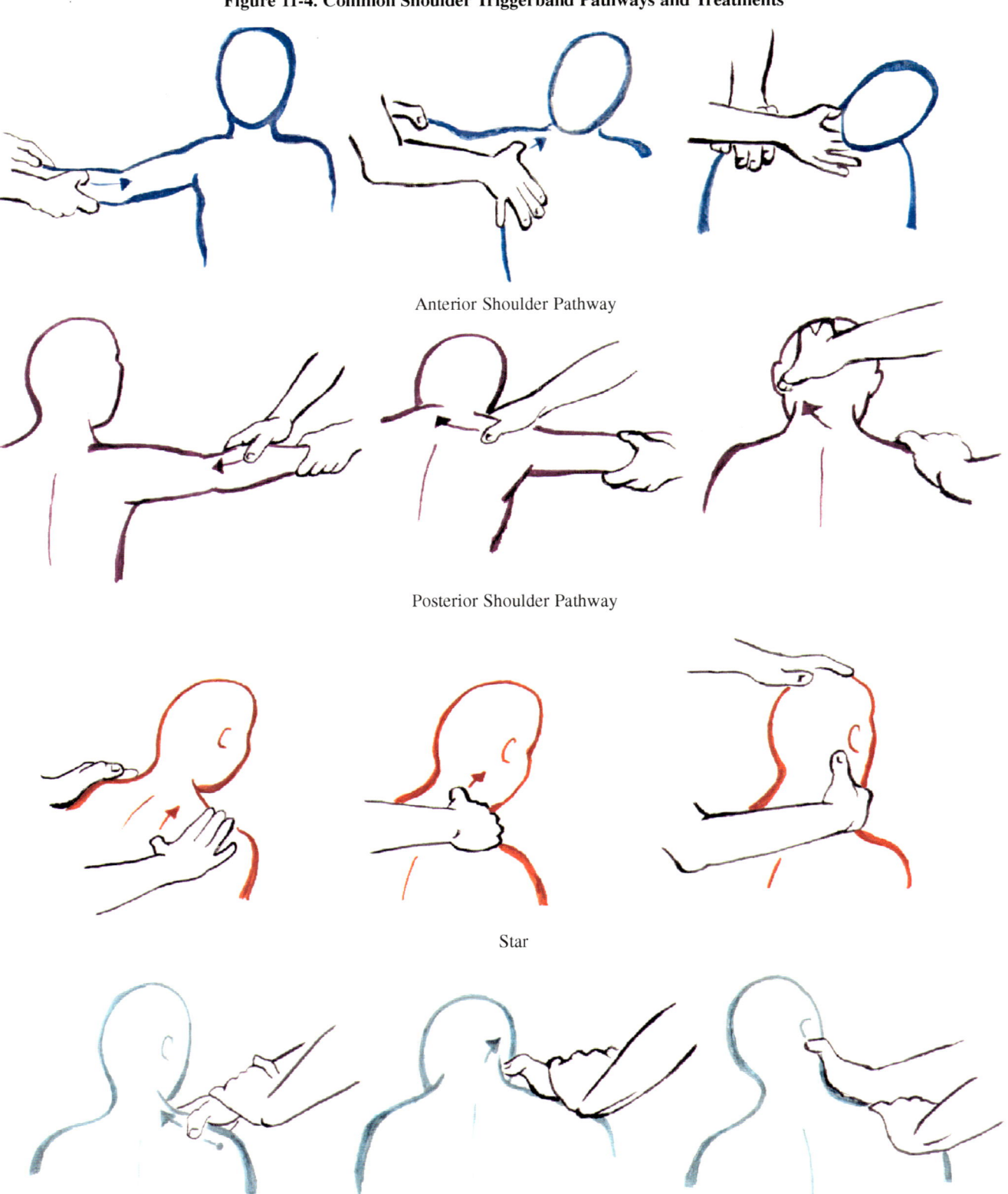

Anterior Shoulder Pathway

Posterior Shoulder Pathway

Star

Shoulder to Mastoid (upper trapezius)

Figure 11-5. Treatment of Supraclavicular Herniated Triggerpoint

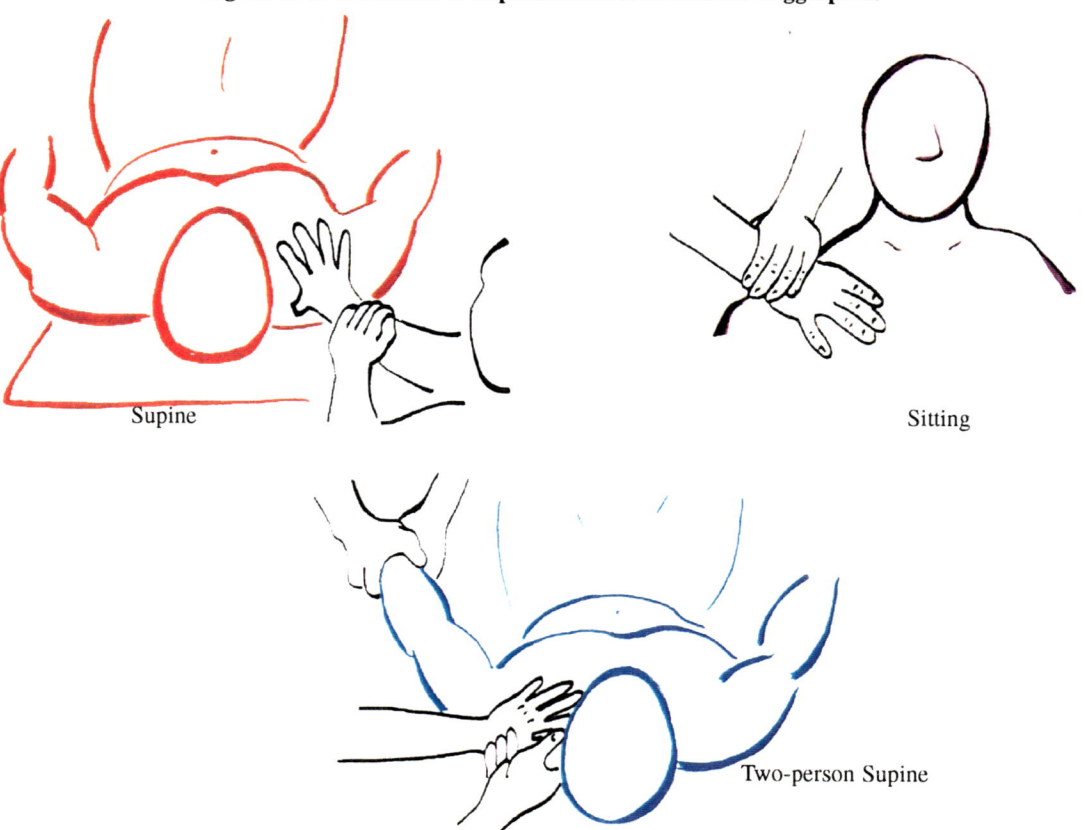

Supine

Sitting

Two-person Supine

Figure 11-6. Continuum Technique of the Shoulder

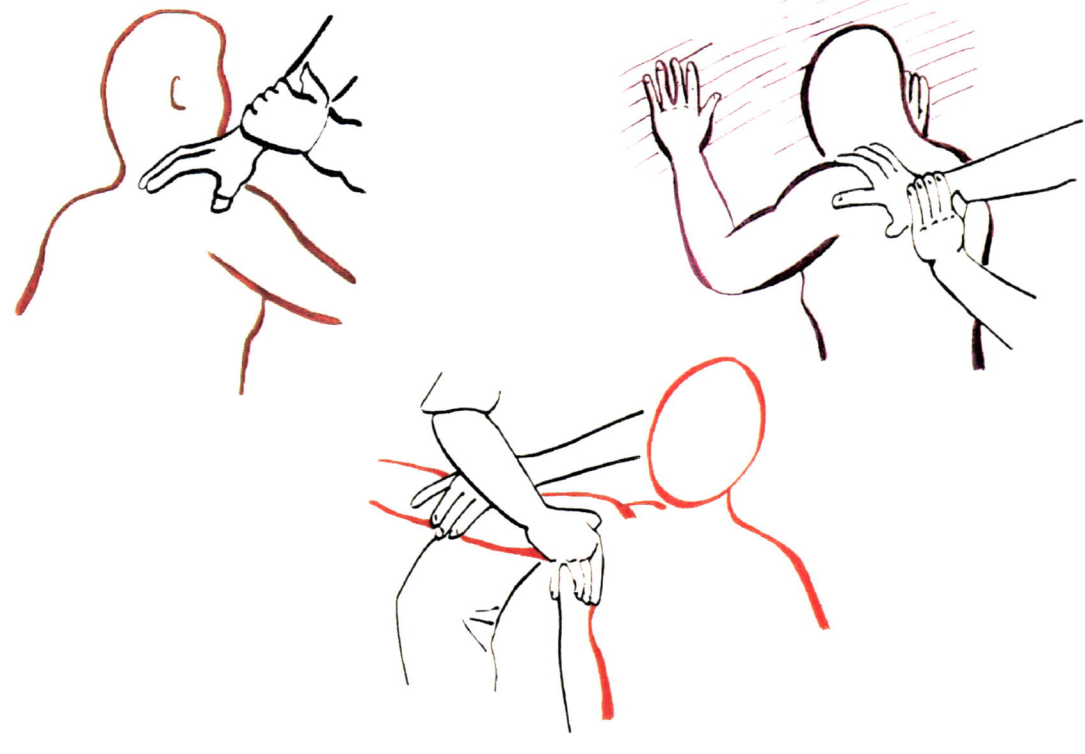

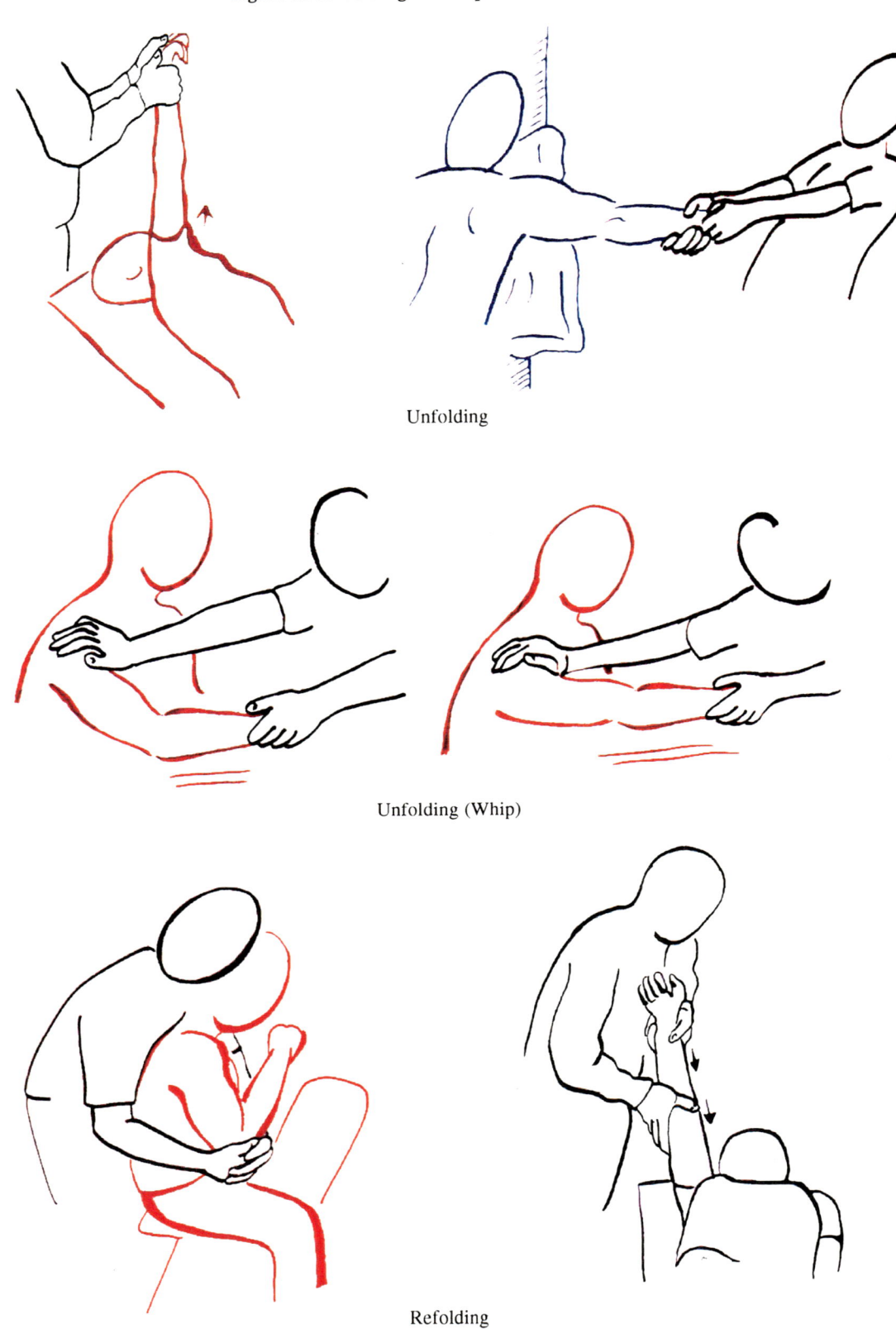

Figure 11-7. Folding Techniques of the Shoulder

Unfolding

Unfolding (Whip)

Refolding

108

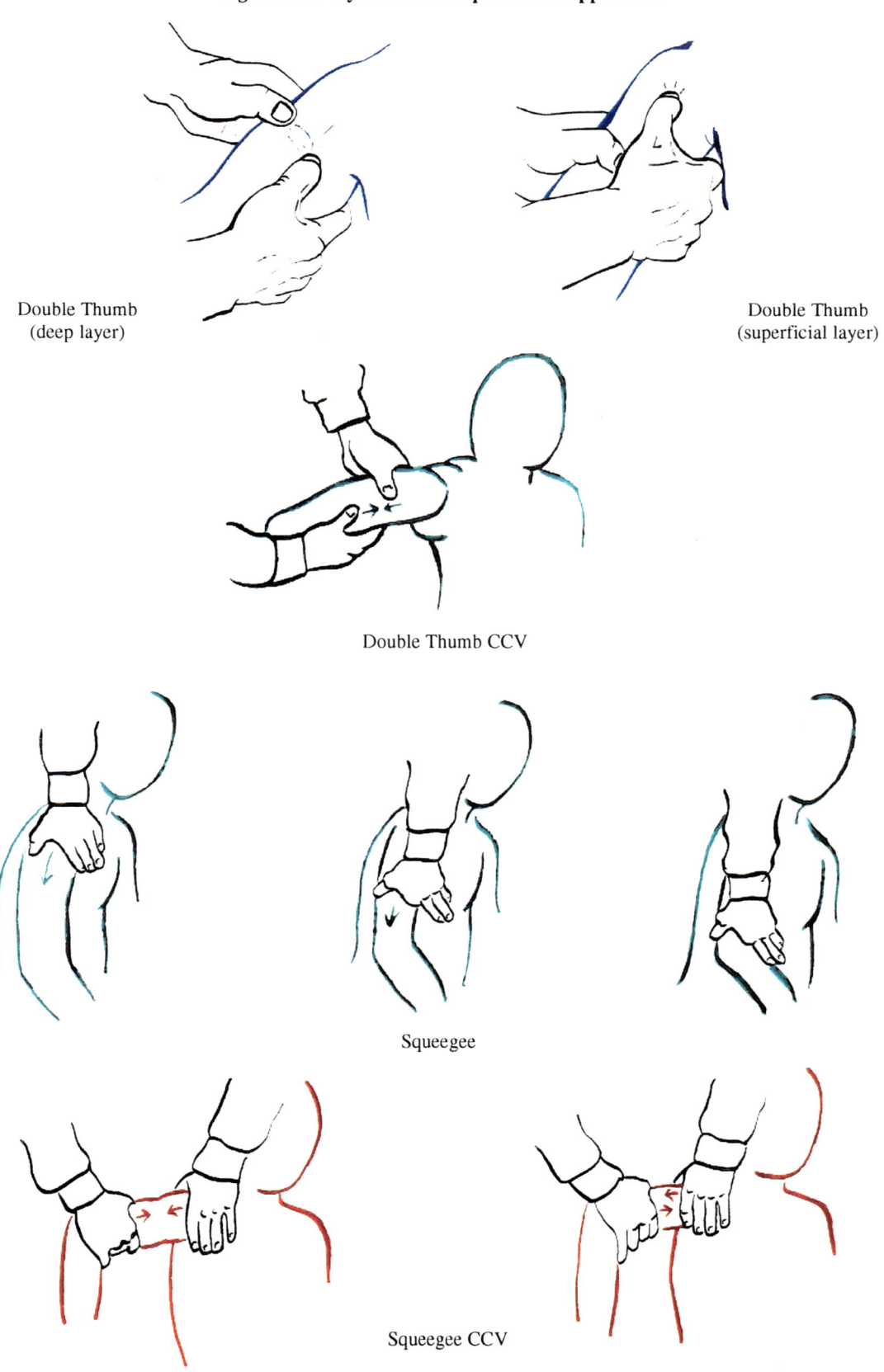

Figure 11-8. Cylinder Techniques of the Upper Arm

Double Thumb (deep layer)

Double Thumb (superficial layer)

Double Thumb CCV

Squeegee

Squeegee CCV

Figure 11-9. Tectonic Techniques of the Shoulder

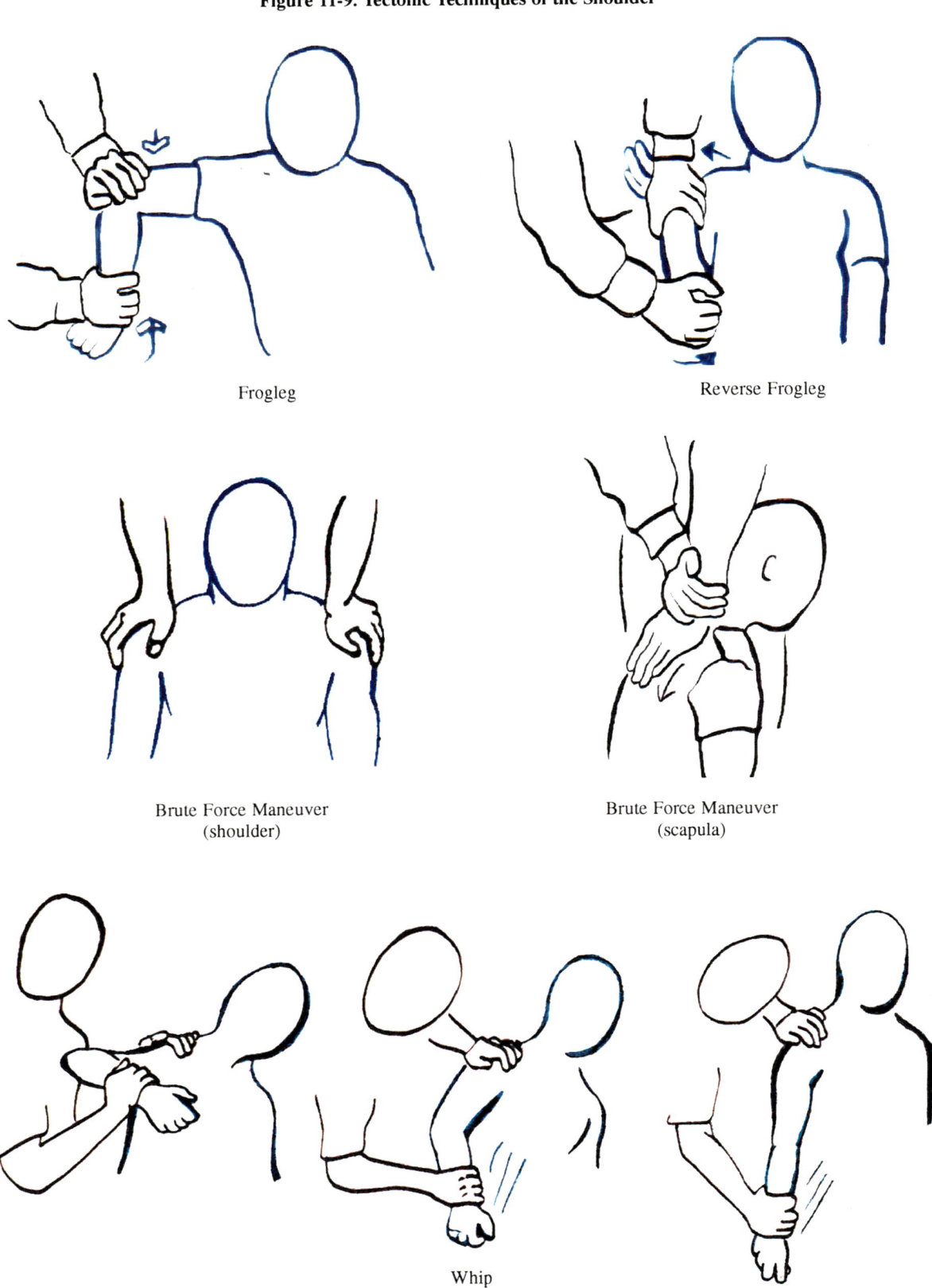

Frogleg

Reverse Frogleg

Brute Force Maneuver
(shoulder)

Brute Force Maneuver
(scapula)

Whip

Chapter 12

THE ORTHOPATHIC TREATMENT OF ANKLE SPRAINS

Orthopedically, sprained ankles are classified by the amount of tearing of the involved ligament, which from the orthopathic perspective is considered to be clinically irrelevant since it neither influences the treatment choices nor is indicative of the anatomical distortion. Although the traditional treatment regimen of wrapping, splinting, crutching, resting, and medicating may reduce discomfort by making the ankle non-functional, the anatomical injury is still present. Take away the crutches, splints, wraps, and medicines and you have the same injured ankle.

Orthopathically, all acutely sprained ankles are differentiated into three kinds: continuum, triggerband, and folding. All three of these ankle sprain types may initially appear to be identical (i.e., they all present with swelling, ecchymosis, tenderness, loss of dorsiflexion, pain with motion, limping gait, and inability to bear weight). However, there are very real differences between them which are highly predictive in determining the success of specific treatment options.

MECHANISM OF INJURY

Every sprained ankle patient will, with proper prodding, reveal a history of injury that is consistent with one of three general mechanisms. The first is eversion of the ankle (with accompanying inversion of the foot). These patients relate that the ankle suddenly buckled outward and they experienced immediate pain. This is the most common history associated with an ankle sprain and is clinically consistent with the physical findings of a *continuum sprained ankle*. An easy way to remember this mechanism of injury is by imagining the most common specific history that is given, which is stepping off the curb and forcefully supinating the foot. For this reason continuum sprained ankles can be thought of as *stepped off the curb wrong ankle sprains*.

The next most common mechanism of injury encountered in a sprained ankle is that of twisting the ankle as the person falls to the same side. As the ankle is everted and the leg is torqued, triggerbands form from the ankle up into the calf. A common specific history that frequently results in *triggerband sprained ankles* is from falling down the stairs. To help envision these sprained ankles, they can be thought of as *tripped down the stairs ankle sprains*.

The third mechanism of injury that results in a sprained ankle occurs when the foot is held in place while the ankle is suddenly everted or twisted. These forces cause the fascial tissue to unfold and then refold in a contorted condition. The most common history given by patients with *folding sprained ankles** is that someone was standing on their foot when the ankle was hurt. Because of this, folding sprained ankles can be thought of as *stepped on the foot ankle sprains*.

Figure 12-1. Three Types of Ankle Sprains

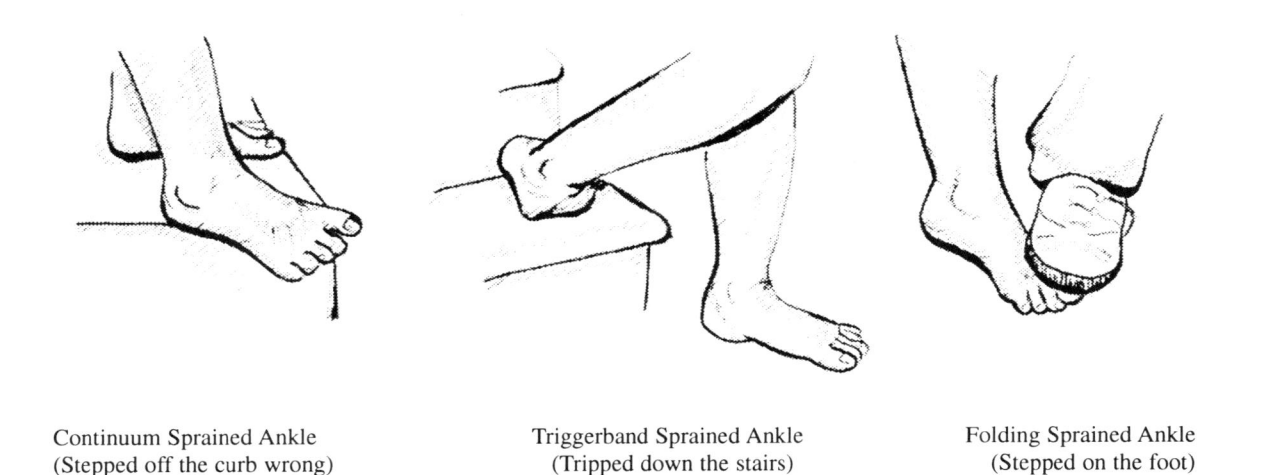

Continuum Sprained Ankle
(Stepped off the curb wrong)

Triggerband Sprained Ankle
(Tripped down the stairs)

Folding Sprained Ankle
(Stepped on the foot)

PATIENTS' DESCRIPTION OF PAIN

Initially an ankle sprain victim will say that the ankle hurts *all over*. But when detail is insisted upon he or she can give a more specific description of the pain that helps determine the general ankle sprain type. The three ways in which patients typically express their discomfort are:
1. Pointing with one finger to specific locations of pain and saying, "The ankle hurts in one (or more) spot(s)"
2. The hand is brought from the ankle up the leg with a sweeping motion – this may be verbalized as, "It pulls into the calf"
3. "It hurts deep in the joint"– watch for the body language of gently wrapping the fingers around the injured ankle, distal leg, or foot

Those patients who complain of pain in one or more spots are describing a continuum sprained ankle. Those who have a pulling pain up the calf will clinically be found to have a triggerband sprained ankle. And those who say they have pain deep in the joint possess a folding sprained ankle.

---

*Note that throughout this text, except where delineated, the term *folding sprained ankles* refers specifically to ankle sprains of the unfolding subtype.

112

Comparing Ankle Sprain Types

Comparative Category	Continuum	Triggerband	Folding
Mechanism of Injury	Eversion of ankle	Eversion of ankle with leg twisting	Eversion or twisting of ankle with foot held in place
Common Hx of Injury	Stepped off curb wrong	Tripped down stairs	Fell with someone standing on foot
Description of Pain	Pain in one or more spots	Pulling pain up calf	Pain deep in joint
Typical Location of Swelling	Lateral ankle	Lateral ankle	Lateral and medial ankle
Frequency	Most common	Less common	Least common
Primary Etiology	Continuum Distortions	Triggerbands	Folding Distortions
Treatment	Continuum Technique	Triggerband Technique	Folding Technique

PHYSICAL FINDINGS OF ANKLE SPRAINS

All sprained ankles present with swelling, pain, and loss of motion. Some patients can walk, some can't. Of those that can walk, few can walk without a limp and very few can run without pain. And sprained ankles of every type contain a continuum distortion in the anterior ankle at the origin or insertion of the anterior tibiofibular ligament. This fascial distortion is the primary cause of diminished dorsiflexion, and because it occurs in every ankle sprain, every sprained ankle should initially receive continuum technique. Once the anterior ankle continuum distortion has been corrected, the ankle sprain is differentiated into its general orthopathic type and the appropriate treatment technique is selected.

On physical exam, continuum ankle sprains have tender spots on the lateral ankle. These are continuum distortions of the calcaneofibular or anterior talofibular ligaments. Other locations of injury are also possible. However, from a treatment perspective, the particular names are unimportant. What is clinically relevant is the exact palpatory location of each continuum distortion.

Triggerband sprained ankles present with a lateral ankle as sore as in a continuum sprained ankle, but the pain pulls into the calf and there are no exact spots of discomfort. Although on palpation these patients have a large tender triggerband that can be palpated along the lateral leg, few patients are aware of its existence until it is brought to their attention. To locate the lateral ankle triggerband pathway, feel for it along the lateral leg with its starting point at the sock line.

Folding sprained ankles feel tight and have a generalized tenderness. On clinical exam, they exhibit swelling over both the lateral and the medial malleolus. Note that medial ankle swelling is indicative of either a fracture or a folding distortion.

Figure 12-2. Typical Swelling Patterns in Ankle Sprain Types

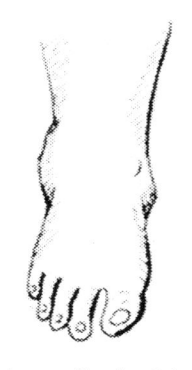

Continuum Sprained Ankle
(lateral swelling)

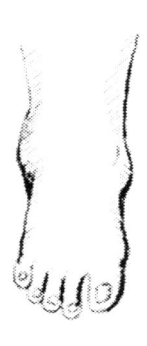

Triggerband Sprained Ankle
(lateral swelling)

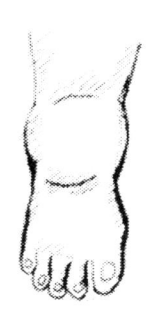

Folding Sprained Ankle
(lateral and medial swelling)

TREATING ANKLE SPRAINS

As stated earlier, the anterior ankle continuum distortion is the first distortion to be treated in every sprained ankle. However, before the actual treatment begins, there are certain assessments that should be made. The first is an orthopedic evaluation to determine the neurovascular supply and the amount of swelling and instability. In addition, the ankle, foot, leg, and any other pertinent areas should be carefully examined. This is especially true if there has been a serious incident in which there is the potential for global injuries, such as from a motorcycle accident.

Once satisfied with the initial physical exam, an x-ray should be considered. If it is negative, then the ankle is orthopathically evaluated and the amount of disability and loss of motion quantified. It is clinically useful to record the amount of dorsiflexion, eversion, and inversion the ankle has, and whether the patient can walk without a limp, stand alone on the injured foot, or walk on the toes or heels. Determine if he/she can bear weight or ambulate on the lateral foot (i.e., walk on the sides of the feet). Can he or she jump or run? Documenting motions and ambulatory abilities (or inabilities) before and after the treatment gives clear and conclusive evidence of a successful (or unsuccessful) treatment outcome.

To assist in evaluating the injured ankle, a grading system can be used to quantify motion and speed. For instance, if dorsiflexion of the injured ankle is one-fourth total motion compared to the opposite ankle, it is graded a *one*. If the speed of dorsiflexion is one-half compared to the other ankle, this is graded a *two*. If the ankle can't dorsiflex at all, it is a *zero*, and if it is the same as the uninjured ankle, it is a *four*. By the same token, three-fourths motion is judged a *three*. If after correcting the anterior ankle continuum distortion, the dorsiflexion has improved from zero to a two, then the treatment was incomplete and strongly suggests a second anterior ankle continuum distortion is present. If this is the case, then it should also be treated.

Figure 12-3. Ankle Sprains of All Three Types Demonstrate Decreased Dorsiflexion

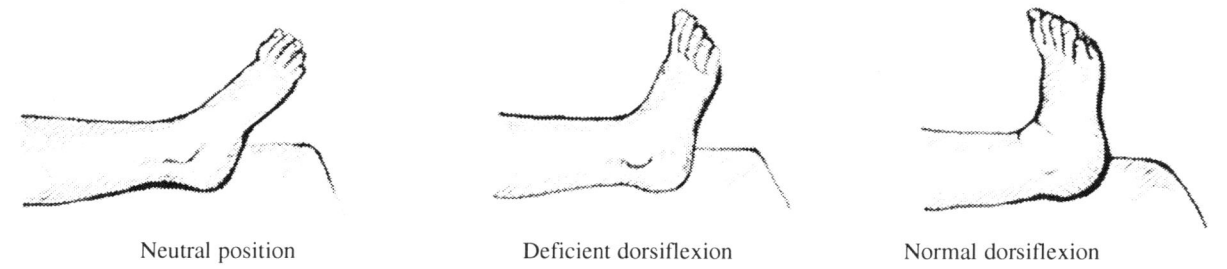

Neutral position   Deficient dorsiflexion   Normal dorsiflexion

The anterior ankle continuum distortion is always the first distortion treated in every sprained ankle. The reason for this is that virtually every sprained ankle has loss of dorsiflexion from this particular distortion. During the ankle exam, this deficit of motion should be brought to the attention of the patient and its ramifications emphasized. It is helpful to explain that loss of dorsiflexion means the ankle can't bend properly, and therefore they can't walk normally.

Before treating the anterior ankle continuum distortion, you may wish to discuss the treatment with the patient and express that it will induce a temporary but significant amount of discomfort. Or you may consider the *quick victory strategy* in which the correction is made so rapidly that the patient believes it is still part of the exam. Be sure to check dorsiflexion immediately after this initial procedure so that the patient can appreciate the change. Typically the results are so dramatically impressive that the patient will be eagerly encouraging you to continue on with the treatment.

The anterior ankle continuum distortion is palpated in the front of the ankle just where the ankle bends (see Figure 12-4 and glossary term *Anterior Ankle Continuum Distortion*). The distortion is normally quite tender and almost feels like a small vitamin gel-cap, i.e., it is firm, but has some give to it. The patient is best positioned for the treatment lying supine with the toes pointed toward the ceiling. (An alternate position is seated with the foot resting on the floor.) The non-treating hand is used to hold the ankle in a position of slight dorsiflexion as the tip of the treating thumb palpates the continuum distortion.

Once the distortion is clearly identified, the direction of force is determined by either palpation or by asking the patient if the thumb has found the spot of most intense discomfort. If the thumb is slightly to the side of the distortion, the firmness will not be centralized below it. To the patient it will feel as if *you're off it*, or *you're next to it*.

Continuum technique is performed by applying a focused force directly into the center of the continuum distortion with the tip of the treating thumb. The force from the thumb is constant and should maximize the patient's discomfort. Pressure is held until the release, which is felt as a sudden lessening of pain by the patient, and as a sudden lessening in firmness of the periosteum by the physician (think of the button slipping into the buttonhole analogy).

The release of a continuum distortion occurs as the osseous components that were stuck in the transition zone between ligament and bone suddenly shift back into the bone. With an experienced orthopath, the entire time involved in treating this distortion may be only five seconds, but for those with less experience, it may take several minutes to properly palpate and align the forces. As with all continuum distortions, the success of the treatment is all-or-none. If it released, the correction was made. If it didn't release, nothing happened. If you are unsure if the correction was made, recheck dorsiflexion. Restoration of this motion is strongly suggestive of a successful procedure.

Not uncommonly, two anterior ankle continuum distortions are present. This is clinically appreciated when the distortion is treated but dorsiflexion is only partially improved. If that is the case, then the second distortion should be palpated and corrected in the same fashion.

Once the anterior ankle continuum distortion is corrected and dorsiflexion is restored, then other distortions are addressed. Note that it is advisable to have already made a decision as to which ankle sprain type is present, for otherwise the wrong technique may be utilized with no possibility of a successful outcome.

Orthopathic Flow Chart of the Acutely Sprained Ankle

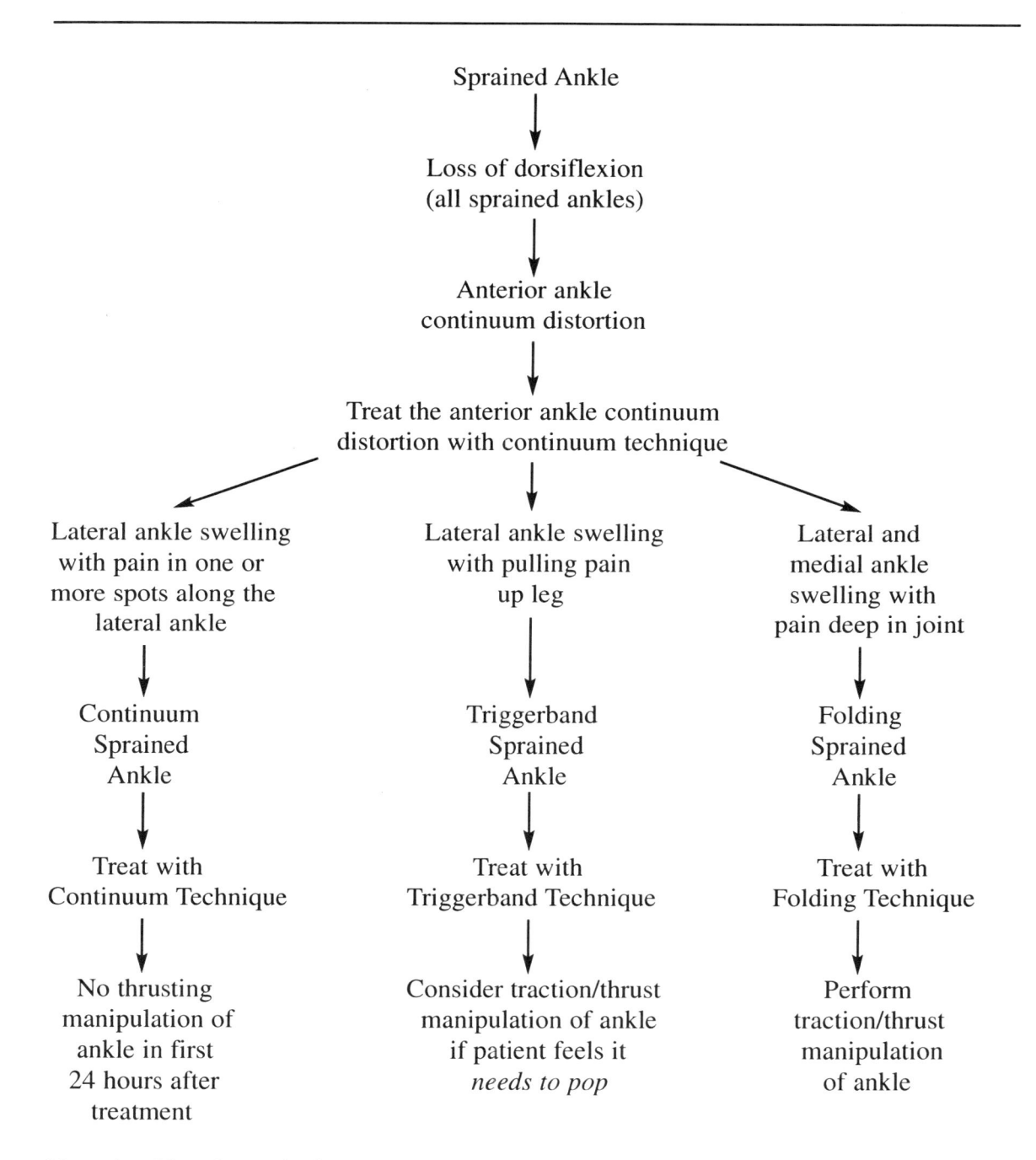

```
                    Sprained Ankle
                          │
                          ▼
                  Loss of dorsiflexion
                  (all sprained ankles)
                          │
                          ▼
                   Anterior ankle
                  continuum distortion
                          │
                          ▼
              Treat the anterior ankle continuum
              distortion with continuum technique
           ┌──────────────┼──────────────┐
           ▼              ▼              ▼
  Lateral ankle swelling  Lateral ankle swelling  Lateral and
  with pain in one or     with pulling pain       medial ankle
  more spots along the    up leg                  swelling with
  lateral ankle                                   pain deep in joint
           │              │              │
           ▼              ▼              ▼
       Continuum       Triggerband      Folding
       Sprained        Sprained         Sprained
       Ankle           Ankle            Ankle
           │              │              │
           ▼              ▼              ▼
       Treat with      Treat with       Treat with
       Continuum       Triggerband      Folding Technique
       Technique       Technique
           │              │              │
           ▼              ▼              ▼
     No thrusting    Consider traction/thrust   Perform
     manipulation of  manipulation of ankle     traction/thrust
     ankle in first   if patient feels it       manipulation
     24 hours after   needs to pop              of ankle
     treatment
```

Note that if at the end of the treatment there is a diffuse pain over the ankle or foot and the patient has worn a splint, consider cylinder technique.

CONTINUUM SPRAINED ANKLES

Continuum ankle sprains are always of the everted subtype and are the most common of the three ankle sprain types (by far). As stated previously, they have spots of pain that are mostly present on the lateral ankle. Treatment consists of first correcting the anterior ankle continuum distortion to restore dorsiflexion, and then correcting the lateral ankle continuum distortions (there may be anywhere from one to five).

Lateral ankle continuum distortions are treated the same way as any other continuum distortions, i.e., the painful joint is gently glided into the position in which it was originally hurt and force equal to that which caused the injury is applied into the distorted transition zone (see Figure 5-2). In the ankle, this means gently everting the ankle and applying focused force with the treating thumb into the spots of most discomfort and holding until release. The most common locations of lateral ankle continuum distortions are the origin and insertion of the talofibular and calcaneofibular ligaments, but other sites do commonly occur.

Once all of the continuum distortions are corrected, the patient is expected to be able to walk without a limp and to have little or no pain. (Note that some patients will be able to run without pain but this is not considered to be the goal of the initial treatment.) Following the treatment ice soaks are encouraged and re-check the next day is recommended for those patients with an incomplete result or those who waited more than three days to seek care.

Figure 12-4. Continuum Technique of the Ankle

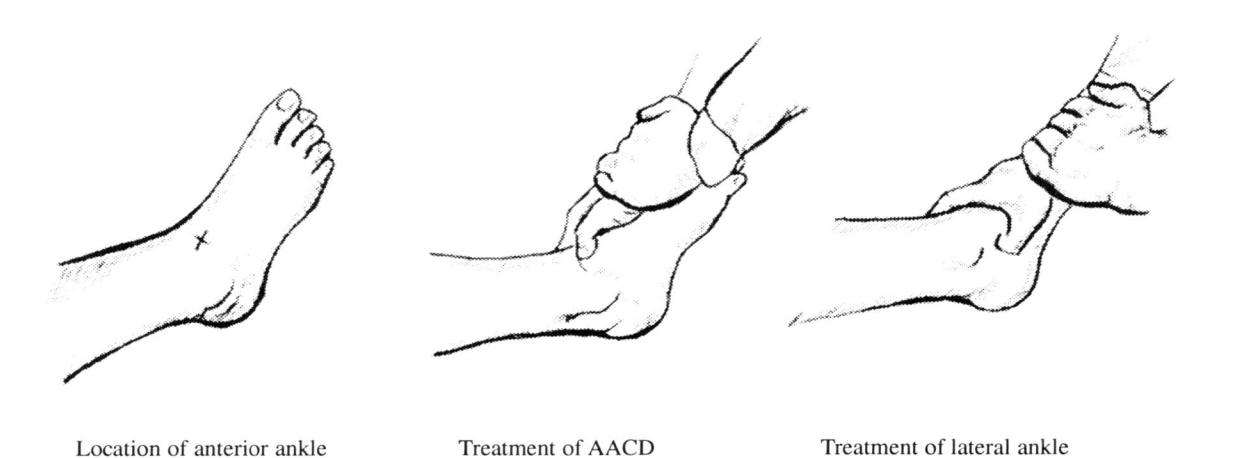

Location of anterior ankle continuum distortion (AACD)

Treatment of AACD

Treatment of lateral ankle continuum distortion

Typical Steps in Treating a Continuum Sprained Ankle

1. Physical examination – record range of motion (passively and actively measure dorsiflexion, eversion and inversion) and check for ligamental instability and vascular compromise.

2. X-ray the ankle to rule out fracture.

3. Explain to the patient that the treatment will cause a temporary increase in discomfort.

4. Restore dorsiflexion by treating the anterior ankle continuum distortion. This is best done with the patient supine and the foot slightly dorsiflexed. Recheck dorsiflexion after treatment.

5. Treat the lateral ankle continuum distortions with continuum technique. Do this by gently rotating the ankle into the position in which it was injured (evert the ankle by rolling it laterally), and with the tip of the thumb, palpate the lateral continuum distortions. Select the most painful distortion. Apply constant and increasing force into the most tender portion of it and hold until it releases.

6. Recheck eversion and inversion. If there is not a dramatic improvement, then palpate for a second or third lateral continuum distortion. Gently guide the ankle into the position of pain (usually eversion), palpate for the most painful spot, and feel for the distortion. Treat with continuum technique, then recheck passive and active eversion and inversion. Repeat the sequence until the patient reports only a diffuse sensation of generalized tenderness or has no pain.

7. Ask the patient to stand and point to where the ankle still hurts. While the patient is standing, correct the distortion in the same manner as previously described. Repeat this step until the patient can stand with little or no pain.

8. Next have the patient walk and identify what movement induces pain. Hold the ankle in that position and correct the distortion.

9. Once the range of motion has been restored and the patient can walk without a limp, the treatment is complete. At home frequent ice/water soaks are suggested and heat (including hot showers or baths) is to be avoided. Crutches and splints are typically unnecessary, and pain medicines are considered to be optional.

10. Follow-up the next day is advisable.

For some patients who are athletes, walking without pain and being limp-free are not enough. These patients may need to get back in the game either the same day or soon. If that is the situation, the treatment can be taken one step further by having him or her run, stopping the ankle in the exact part of the gait that causes pain, and then treating with the ankle held in that position. This process should be repeated until the athlete can run without pain. Note that residual continuum distortions may occur in other portions of the ankle, or on the bottom of the foot, so you may have to listen and palpate carefully to find them. If after all that, the athlete still can't run without pain, look for other fascial distortion types or re-treat in 24 hours.

TRIGGERBAND SPRAINED ANKLES

Triggerband sprained ankles appear clinically to be almost identical to continuum sprained ankles in that there is loss of dorsiflexion, lateral ankle swelling, ecchymosis, pain, and limping gait (if the patient can walk at all). The differences between the two are, of course, mechanism of injury, patient's description of the pain pattern, physical palpatory findings, and the success of using triggerband technique rather than continuum technique. This final difference between the two cannot be stressed enough — these are two distinct etiologies of ankle sprains and using the wrong technique will always result in failure.

As stated earlier, triggerband ankle sprains are less common than their continuum counterparts. Still, they make up a large enough portion of the total number of ankle sprains that they are commonly encountered in the emergency room setting or in a busy sports medicine practice. And fortunately, the dramatic treatment results that so often occur with continuum ankle sprains also are expected with triggerband ankle sprains.

In treating triggerband sprained ankles, the initial evaluation is identical to continuum sprained ankles. Just as with continuum injuries, the anterior ankle continuum distortion is treated first. Once this is corrected, the involved triggerbands are located and treated.

The most important ankle sprain triggerband of all is found on the lateral lower leg with its starting point at the sock level. It is treated by having the thumb push inferiorly (down the leg), to the ankle, then around and below the lateral malleolus, onto the dorsal foot, and finally to either a distal metatarsal or to the end of one of the toes (fourth and fifth are the most common). Note that this pathway is present in virtually every triggerband sprained ankle.

This *lateral ankle triggerband* is, at times, a teaching workshop for the entire triggerband concept. For it is here, along this pathway, that so often the patient's pain can be moved from one location to another. If the orthopath pushes the twist down the ankle and leaves it on the foot, the patient may complain of foot pain. If the twist is moved back behind the lateral malleolus, he or she will have ankle pain, and if the twist is forced into the calf, the complaint is of calf pain. Wherever the twist is moved to is where the patient will have pain. For this reason, it is necessary to correct the triggerband along its entire course from the lateral leg, through the ankle, onto the foot, to the end of the affected toe. Although not every patient with a triggerband sprained ankle will demonstrate this movement of pain so clearly, it is a common clinical finding and is pathognomonic of a triggerband sprained ankle.

Figure 12-5. Triggerband Technique of the Lateral Ankle Pathway

Starting point is on the lateral ankle at the sock line.

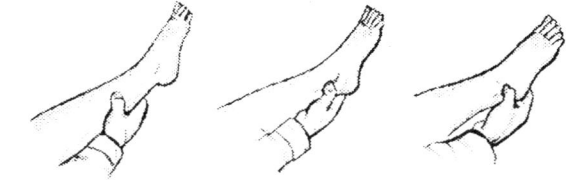

The pathway continues inferiorly. . .and courses behind the lateral malleolus. . .

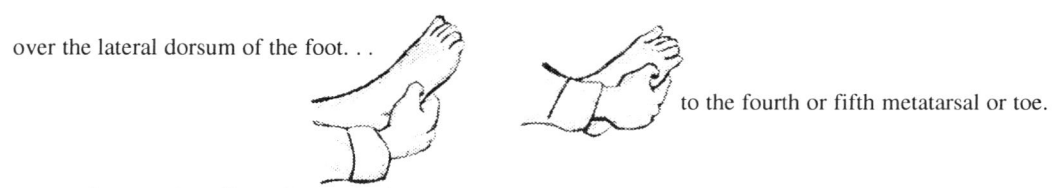

over the lateral dorsum of the foot. . .

to the fourth or fifth metatarsal or toe.

In most patients, the direction of triggerband technique should be inferior (i.e., toward the foot), but a small number of patients benefit little from this direction. If the technique was properly applied and the diagnosis is relatively certain, and yet the treatment was only partially effective, consider changing directions and pushing the triggerband from the foot up into the calf to the sock line (think of the Ziploc® bag being zipped closed).

Although the lateral ankle triggerband pathway is the most common ankle triggerband, several other pathways may also be present in the same patient. These triggerbands run parallel to the lateral ankle triggerband but are either more anterior or posterior. If they are present, treat them as well.

One big difference between a completed triggerband sprained ankle treatment and a continuum sprained ankle treatment is the sensation of tightness the patient may still have in the ankle. Triggerband patients may say something to the effect that the ankle *feels like it needs to pop*, meaning that there is a small folding distortion present in the ankle capsule. Even though this person may have had an excruciatingly tender ankle only a few minutes before, it is generally okay to attempt a gentle traction/thrust manipulation of the ankle. To manipulate the ankle, the patient is placed in the supine position and holds onto the head end of the exam table with his or her outstretched hands (so he/she isn't pulled during the treatment). The ankle is dorsiflexed and traction is maintained. Then a swift but smooth pulling force is introduced into the ankle. When performed properly, a pop is felt or heard.

However, it should be made clear — never manipulate a continuum sprained ankle on the initial treatment because you will reverse all of the hard work that you have done and the patient will act as if the ankle has been suddenly re-sprained!

Typical Steps in Treating a Triggerband Sprained Ankle

1. Physical examination – record passive and active range of motion and check for ligamental instability and vascular compromise.

2. X-ray the ankle to rule out fracture.

3. Explain to the patient that there will be a temporary increase in discomfort.

4. Ask the patient to show where the pain is. Note that he/she typically will make a sweeping motion with his or her fingers along the triggerband pathway from the calf onto the foot.

5. Emphasize the loss of dorsiflexion, then treat the anterior ankle continuum distortion with continuum technique. Recheck dorsiflexion. Emphasize the motion again so that he/she appreciates the improvement.

6. Palpate along the sock line for the starting point of the lateral ankle triggerband pathway. Once found, treat the triggerband from superior to inferior. Note that it ends at or near the base of the toes (fourth and fifth are most common). Before and after this treatment, check eversion and inversion.

7. Recheck motion. If not improved, either re-treat the same pathway, search for other pathways, or consider reversing the direction of treatment.

8. Once dorsiflexion, inversion, and eversion are normalized, have the patient stand and determine areas of pain. Find the remaining triggerbands and treat while the patient is standing.

9. Once the patient can stand pain-free, have him/her walk. If there is still pain, locate and treat the residual triggerbands.

10. If the patient feels as if the ankle needs to be popped (most have very strong feelings on this), then use traction/thrust manipulation.

11. Frequent ice/water soaks are encouraged, splints and crutches should be unnecessary, pain medicines are optional, and recheck is advised the next day for those with less than an optimal result.

Folding Sprained Ankles

Folding ankle sprains are the least frequently encountered of the three types of ankle sprains. However, in certain athletic events such as hockey and basketball, they are seen not too uncommonly. Hockey and basketball not only produce many ankle injuries, but also have more than their share of ankle sprains with someone standing or falling on the foot during the accident.

Note that in folding ankle sprains, lateral ankle swelling is always present and medial swelling is *almost always* present. However, it should be remembered that as a general rule, medial ankle swelling is indicative of either a folding sprained ankle or an ankle fracture. And as with the other two types, foot dorsiflexion is always impaired and is the result of the anterior ankle continuum distortion. Again, as with continuum and triggerband ankle sprains, this distortion is treated first. Once dorsiflexion is restored, the focus of the treatment then centers on eliminating folding distortions.

To treat the misfolded fascial tissue around the ankle, the ankle itself must be tractioned. To apply traction, the patient is placed supine on the exam table with the knee extended. The physician, who is standing at the foot of the table, introduces gentle dorsiflexion into the ankle. The treating hands are wrapped around the midfoot and the fingers are intertwined. The foot is slowly lifted up off the table at a 10° to 30° angle as traction is introduced into the joint capsule (this is best done by having the physician extend the elbows and roll back on his/her heels). Traction is steadily increased until a release is felt. The release may be subtle (and feel as only a slight *give*), or more pronounced (and feel like a series of short *clunks*). Note that the entire process of folding technique (i.e., traction, unfolding, and refolding) can take as little as several seconds or as long as several minutes.

Figure 12-6. Folding Technique of the Ankle

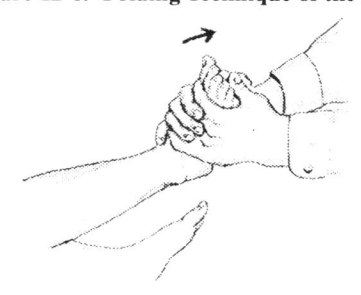

After folding technique is finished, ankle motion is rechecked and compared to its pre-treatment status. If the result is satisfactory, the patient is instructed to stand. If there is pain with standing, this means that residual folding distortions remain and need to be treated. Folding technique is then re-instigated with the patient again in the supine position. This time, the direction of traction is changed to focus the pulling forces into the fascial plane that hasn't completely unfolded. If the patient feels that the ankle "needs to pop" then traction the ankle again and introduce a sharp pulling thrust. Folding technique is repeated several times, with adjustments made in the direction of force until the patient can stand and walk pain-free.

Typical Steps in Treating a Folding Sprained Ankle

1. Physical examination – record passive and active range of motion and check for instability and vascular compromise.

2. X-ray the ankle to rule out fracture.

3. Ask the patient to show with his or her hand where the most discomfort is. (This is usually done by placing the palm gently over the ankle, foot, or distal leg.)

4. Explain to the patient that the first portion of the treatment may be uncomfortable.

5. Treat the anterior ankle continuum distortion. Compare dorsiflexion before and after.

6. Apply traction to the ankle with the patient supine. Intertwine the fingers around the midfoot and extend the elbows as you lean back on your heels to allow the weight of your body to pull the ankle towards you. Constant steady force will help unfold the distorted fascia and allow it to refold into its uninjured configuration.

7. Repeat step 6, but slightly alter the direction of force so that the correction can be focused into the residual painful areas.

8. Repeat step 7, but have the patient standing when determining the residual painful areas (treat again in the supine position).

9. Repeat step 8, but have the patient walking when determining residual painful areas (treat again in the supine position).

10. Traction/thrust manipulation should then be instigated. This procedure is performed in much the same way as folding traction, except that a quick pulling thrust is initiated to more forcefully unfold the ankle capsule. When this procedure is properly performed, a *clunk* or *pop* is heard.

11. Once the patient can walk without limping and has little or no discomfort, the treatment is considered to be completed.

12. Frequent ice/water soaks are suggested, crutches and splints should be unnecessary, and pain medications are optional. Recheck in 24 hours and re-treat if needed.

Refolding Sprained Ankles

Refolding sprained ankles are uncommon and occur when the ankle is jammed or compressed against the ground or other structure. They generally present in much the same manner as unfolding sprained ankles in that there is bi-malleolar swelling accompanied with the verbal description of discomfort of aching deep in the joint. And just as with unfolding sprained ankles, the corresponding body language tends to be a gentle wrapping of the fingers around the distal leg, ankle, or foot. However, refoldings differ from unfoldings in three important ways:

1. Mechanism of injury
2. Additional body language – rubbing fingers back and forth across anterior ankle
3. Treatment – compression/thrust of the heel into the leg

Combination Sprained Ankles

Although most ankle sprains can be easily broken down into the three categories of continuum, triggerband, and folding, some patients present with injuries containing two or all three fascial distortion types (i.e., lateral ankle continuum distortions, triggerbands, and folding distortions). The treatment of *combination sprained ankles* is essentially the same as previously described. First, treat the anterior ankle continuum distortion to restore dorsiflexion, then treat either the folding distortion or the lateral ankle triggerband. And finally treat the lateral ankle continuum distortions. (There may be some palpatory confusion in distinguishing between triggerbands and continuum distortions; but remember triggerbands move and continuum distortions release.) Do not manipulate the joint on the initial treatment. Note that combination injuries occur when the ankle encounters a combination of forces at the time of injury, and typically respond just as well to FDM treatments as non-combination ankle sprains.

Cylinder Sprained Ankles

Although cylinder distortions are commonly found in foot sprains (along with triggerbands, continuum distortions, and folding distortions), they are rarely diagnosed in ankle sprains. And when involved, they are practically never the initial cause of injury but instead result from splinting. It seems that the longer an ankle splint is worn, the more likely it is that a cylinder distortion occurs. The best approach to cylinder ankle sprains is prevention. This is done by avoiding the use of ankle splints altogether. However, if another doctor has already applied a splint, or if for whatever reason its use seems appropriate, then the length of time it is worn should be minimized.

Clinically, treatment of cylinder distortions in the ankle is initiated after all the other fascial distortions have been corrected. The double thumb cylinder technique is the preferred method, not the Indian burn technique which in the foot and ankle has a tendency to create more cylinder distortions than it corrects.

The symptomatic areas are treated with firm but gentle opposing traction from the physician's thumbs. The deep layer is treated first so that the traction is perpendicular to the bones (i.e., one thumb is pulling laterally while the other is pulling medially). Then the superficial layer is treated. The thumb traction is then parallel to the bones, so one thumb pulls up and the other down.

Remember that cylinder distortions are notorious for the pain *jumping* from one area to another, so don't be frustrated if this occurs. Treat each tangled coil one at a time and recheck the patient the next day.

TREATMENT FAILURES

Of all the injuries treated with the orthopathic approach, ankle sprains indubitably have the highest success rate. This is because the anatomy in the ankle is easy to palpate and the distortions are literally right at the treating doctor's fingertips. Another positive contributing factor is that most ankle sprain patients are highly motivated to accept the treatment because the orthopedic alternative of splinting and crutches is generally considered to be undesirable. Unfortunately, inexperienced physicians will at first have failures or partial successes. The reasons are shown below in decreasing order of likelihood:

1. *Failure to properly diagnose* the orthopathic type of ankle sprain. When this occurs the treatment will fail because the proper technique was not employed.

2. *Failure to use adequate force* – an ankle sprain is a painful injury and some physicians hesitate in applying necessary force (especially critical in treating continuum sprained ankles).

3. *Application of heat* – prior to being seen, the patient has taken a warm shower or soaked the ankle in hot water. This will negate the subjective benefit of the treatment and result in a much more painful therapy.

4. A *fracture* exists that wasn't appreciated on x-ray.

To become skilled at the orthopathic treatment of ankle sprains requires the physician to be strongly motivated to succeed. But in addition to that, he or she must be willing to experience and experiment, and to take responsibility for treatment failures as well as successes. Perhaps in no other injury treated with fascial distortion techniques is the difference between success and failure so strongly demarcated.

Chapter 13

FASCIAL DISTORTION TECHNIQUES IN THE EMERGENCY ROOM

Fascial distortion techniques provide emergency room physicians with non-invasive modalities which when properly utilized, demonstrate objective, clear-cut, and immediate results. In the case of whiplash injury, for example, the elimination of symptoms and restoration of cervical motion not only benefits the patient but also clinically confirms the diagnosis. In addition, the success of the treatment underscores the implausibility of serious secondary injuries (such as a fracture) being concurrently present. And since the objective post-treatment findings are easily documented, they add credence to the contention that quality care was delivered. Starting from the head down, the most commonly encountered fascial injuries seen in the Emergency Department are discussed, along with their treatments.

HEADACHES

Headaches are one of the most common complaints seen in the ER. Once an organic etiology is ruled out, an orthopathic interpretation can be considered. Perhaps the best headache candidates to receive FDM techniques are those with a *pulling* or *burning* pain from the upper back or neck. Note again that the words pulling or burning signify that that the underlying etiology is a triggerband. The two most prominent headache triggerbands, the *star* and the *upper trapezius*, are differentiated from each other by the patient's body language (a sweeping motion with fingers from upper back to mastoid for the star, and a sweeping motion from shoulder to mastoid for the upper trapezius). In either case, triggerband technique is performed along the involved pathway. Be advised that with star headaches, the fascial fibers are often twisted along the pathway in the peri-occipital region, so extra force is needed at the base of the skull to make the correction.

One-sided headaches with the head tilted to the side of pain are often the result of the supraclavicular herniated triggerpoint (SCHTP). The main symptom of this headache is an ache and tightness along the entire side of the affected neck, face, and head. Treatment consists of herniated triggerpoint therapy in which the SCHTP is first located and then treated with force from the physician's thumb. The goal of the therapy is to push the protruding tissue below the fascial plane. If there is a partial result with the treatment, repeat the procedure with more force and finesse.

One particularly miserable headache is commonly referred to by patients as the *behind-the-eye headache*. The complaint is of a dull but pronounced ache (similar to an ice cream headache of the sinuses) that is located just behind the affected orbit. Physical findings often include photophobia and an inability to open the eyelid fully. Treatment consists of three components:

1. Triggerband technique of the pathway from just anterior to the TMJ along the eyebrow to the lacrimal bone
2. Herniated triggerpoint therapy of the lacrimal herniated triggerpoint
3. Gentle ice massage along the treated areas

Note that the triggerband subtype for this headache is either a *twist* or *grain of salt*. This means that the affected fascial band is very narrow, so only light force is needed for correction. And also care must be taken in correcting the lacrimal HTP. It is the smallest and most delicate herniated triggerpoint in the body so only the tip of the thumb can be used. Remember that it is a tiny HTP and not a continuum distortion, so use petite pressure to coax the protruding tissue below the lacrimal bone.

Other cephalgias include:
- *Migraine-like headaches* in which the patient pushes his/her fingers into the skull sutures – treat with refolding technique of the sutures by literally pushing the bones together. At times a pop may be elicited. Cranial technique can be applied in conjunction with refolding technique to force fluid through the suture joints of these combination refolding/tectonic injuries.
- *Squeezing headaches* in which the patient either describes the discomfort as squeezing, or squeezes the scalp with his/her hands or fingers – treat with double thumb cylinder technique (or double thumb CCV) along the areas of spasm
- *Scalp headaches* with pain along a specific line – treat with triggerband technique along the affected pathway

TEMPOROMANDIBULAR JOINT PAIN

Injured temporomandibular joints possess tiny fascial distortions, which are difficult to palpate and require expertise and finesse to correct. The most common TMJ distortions are triggerbands, continuum distortions, and unfolding and refolding distortions. Triggerband subtypes found along the TMJ are either twists or grains of salt (meaning they are very tiny). TMJ triggerbands often give the sensation of pulling on the jaw, teeth, or neck. The triggerband pathway is determined by knowing where the pain pulls from (most patients have a clear concept of this), and then palpating the distortion. Many of these tiny triggerbands originate on the jaw or temporalis muscle and the patient can point to where the pain begins. The distortion can then be engaged with the tip of the treating thumb. Once found, the triggerband is ironed out along its entire pathway by force from the physician's thumb. If the twist is felt in the temporal area, treat by pushing it down and through the TMJ to the base of the mastoid. If instead it is palpated on the jaw, the pathway will course from the mandible up through the TMJ. From there it continues upward and posteriorly so that it traverses above the ear to the mastoid.

Continuum distortions of the TMJ are tiny and require a good deal of specific force to correct. In many cases, a continuum distortion is being held in place by a nearby triggerband. If so, treat the triggerband first. TMJ continuum distortions are treated by first palpating the exact point of most intense discomfort and then holding firm pressure until release. Often continuum distortions of the TMJ occur deep within the joint, so precise direction and force are necessary for a successful treatment.

Although folding TMJ complaints include aching deep in the joint, unfolding and refolding distortions should be distinguished so the treatment can be specified. Patients with unfolding TMJ's feel as if their jaw doesn't close all the way (treatment is traction/thrust), whereas patients with refolding TMJ's feel as if the jaw doesn't open fully (treatment is compression/thrust). In either case the patient is positioned supine with the doctor at the head-end of the table. The physician's fingers are interlaced around the chin and the palms of the hands cradle the ears. With the mouth slightly open, either a thrusting pull (unfolding) or push (refolding) is directed along the line of the mandible. If the treatment is successful a small pop should be heard or felt.

EAR PAIN

This topic could also be classified as the *ear infection that wasn't*. So many times, patients with so-called earaches have been unsuccessfully treated for various lengths of time with antibiotics and decongestants, yet on exam the ear looks normal and the TMJ is not tender. Although these individuals may think they have an ear infection, in actuality they don't. On palpation the pain is easily reproduced and magnified by applying pressure to the area posterior to the angle of the jaw near the mastoid. In this small fossa sits the rim of the atlas where continuum distortions are common. Treatment with continuum technique is done by applying firm pressure with the tip of the thumb into the fossa. The patient's head should be slightly side-bent and the mouth should be partly open with the jaw relaxed. Firm pressure is increased until release (care should be taken in treating elderly or osteoporotic patients). Even in those patients who have had ear pain for some time, one treatment is usually sufficient to correct the problem.

Another fairly common complaint of ear pain is tightness in the ear itself. This description of discomfort is commonly associated with tectonic fixations of the middle ear bones. Correction is made with a thrusting manipulation of the auricle (grasp it and give a quick yank) which when done properly results in an audible pop. If unsuccessful change the direction of tug.

SEPARATED SHOULDERS (ACROMIOCLAVICULAR SPRAINS)

In a separated shoulder the clavicle has been partially forced away from the scapula at the acromioclavicular joint. In the acute injury, as is commonly seen in the emergency room setting, triggerbands and continuum distortions dominate. Triggerbands cause pain that pull along the clavicle to the shoulder. Begin treating by first palpating the most tender area of the injury. Once it is located, apply firm pressure to feel if it moves or hurts only in that one spot. If it *stays put* then it is a continuum distortion. Treat by holding firm pressure until release. If it can be induced to move, use triggerband technique and follow the distortion along its course. Several triggerbands and continuum distortions are usually present in separated shoulders. The more that are corrected, the greater motion and less pain the patient will have. Even though initially these patients may present to the ER with a high magnitude of pain and immobility, they often respond well and leave the ER with normal range of motion, and only a residual dull ache. And again, ice massage is helpful before and/or after the treatment.

ACUTELY FROZEN SHOULDERS

Acutely frozen shoulders typically respond well to fascial distortion treatments and have an excellent objective and subjective result. Many will respond completely to treatment of the supraclavicular herniated triggerpoint, and correction of the anterior or posterior shoulder triggerband pathways. Since acutely frozen (also called sprained) shoulders typically have only one or a few distortions to correct, they are good injuries on which to begin practicing FDM techniques. The distortions tend to be large and one treatment usually eliminates the injury. Again it is helpful to compare motion before and after the treatment so the patient can appreciate the objective result. The evaluation and treatment of the injured shoulder is discussed in much more detail in the sore shoulder chapter.

UPPER ARM PAIN

Acute pain in the upper arm that is not a fracture, medical, or orthopedic problem tends to be caused by either triggerbands or cylinder distortions. If the pain is pulling, think triggerbands. The most common triggerband involving the upper arm is the anterior shoulder pathway (see Figure 3-3). If the injured arm is cupped with the palm of the opposite hand, think cylinder distortion (see Figure 11-1). These patients often give a history that someone twisted or pulled on their arm. In cylinder injures, the pain is diffuse and difficult to localize. Note that some cylinder sore upper arms present with global loss of motion of the shoulder and have a biting pain upon adduction. Triggerband and cylinder sore shoulders are discussed in Chapter 11.

ELBOW PAIN

Caution should be taken when evaluating any acutely injured elbow with swelling. Radial head fractures are common and are often misdiagnosed; so you may wish to adopt the philosophy that any acutely injured elbow with swelling should initially be considered fractured regardless of what the x-ray shows. Other types of elbow pain include nursemaid's (which responds best to folding/thrusting manipulation), and lateral and medial epicondylitis. In the fascial distortion model epicondylitis, a.k.a. tennis elbow, is viewed as being caused by either triggerbands or continuum distortions.

Triggerband elbow strains produce a pulling pain down the medial or lateral forearm. Treatment consists of first finding the triggerband starting point (the sorest spot on the elbow) and then correcting the fascial band along its entire pathway from the elbow onto the forearm and down to the wrist. Note that most medial elbow triggerbands have a pathway along the medial forearm, and most lateral triggerbands maintain a lateral pathway.

Continuum distortions of the elbow hurt in one or more spots. Treatment consists of flexing the elbow, locating the exact point of maximum discomfort with the tip of the treating thumb, and then applying pressure until the transition zone shifts back into its uninjured configuration.

Cylinder distortions also occur in the acutely injured elbow. Patients with these injuries say, "The elbow hurts all over." The discomfort itself seems to be just below the skin but the exact location can't be localized. The mechanism of injury responsible for elbow cylinder distortion formation is typically a pulling or twisting of the involved extremity. On physical exam, the motion is grossly normal (shoulder internal rotation may be slow or hesitant) and there are no spots of tenderness which when palpated magnify the discomfort. Treatment of choice is Indian burn cylinder technique in which one hand is placed several inches above the elbow, while the other hand is placed several inches below it. Traction is instigated so that the proximal hand pulls toward the shoulder and the distal hand pulls toward the wrist. Once traction is achieved, the upper hand initiates rotation in a clockwise direction, at the same time the lower hand rotates in a counterclockwise direction. The traction and torque are held until the tautness of the tissue diminishes. If the result is less than acceptable, repeat the procedure with the direction of rotation reversed.

Folding distortions are yet another source of elbow pain and hurt deep in the joint. Unfoldings result from a pulling injury (for instance from throwing a bowling ball), whereas refoldings occur from a compression injury (such as falling on an outstretched hand). Treatment consists of traction/thrust for unfoldings (see *Whip*, Figure 11-7) and compression/thrust for refoldings.

Tectonic fixations of the elbow generally lead to the verbal assertion that "the elbow needs to pop." This is the *green light* for employing frogleg and/or reverse frogleg manipulations. The technique is performed essentially the same as for the shoulder (see Figure 11-9) except that the elbow is flexed as much as possible during the thrust. When the treatment is successful, the elbow manipulates with a large pop or clunk.

FOREARM PAIN

The most common diagnosis in acute forearm pain (other than fracture) is tendonitis. In the ER setting, these patients typically give a history that involves a repetitive motion such as several hours of scrubbing the floor or vigorous use of sandpaper. Occasionally the forearm will exhibit warmth or swelling. Hand and wrist motion are generally impaired (sometimes profoundly) and compounding the problem, many patients have exacerbated the injury by applying heating pads or hot wet washcloths. Typically these acute cases of tendonitis respond well to triggerband technique. The responsible triggerbands begin in the proximal forearm and reach into the hand along the course of the flexor and extensor tendons. Treatment is best initiated from the source of pain down the forearm following the involved tendons. A successful result is often dramatic and the patient is immediately able to make a fist, flex and extend the wrist, and move the fingers normally — all without pain.

Continuum distortions in a tendon are less common than triggerbands, but when present cause similar symptoms. The precise location of discomfort in continuum tendonitis is at the origin or insertion of flexor or extensor tendons. The treatment of these injuries is with ice massage or ice/water soaks followed by continuum technique.

Folding distortions of the interosseous membrane between the radius and ulna cause an aching discomfort deep in the forearm and may interfere with supination and pronation. Treatment for unfoldings consists of tractioning and thrusting apart the radius and ulna with the physician's hands and fingers. The refolding correction is accomplished by thrusting the radius and ulna together. In either case, a successful manipulation is accompanied by an audible pop.

WRIST PAIN

Fractures are perhaps the most common type of wrist injury seen in the ER, but patients with contusions, sprains, and carpal tunnel syndrome also come walking through the doors. Anatomically, contusions are continuum distortions of the inverted type and may or may not respond well to continuum technique. To treat, hold the wrist in the position of pain and apply firm pressure with the tip of the thumb directly into the most tender spot until the distortion releases.

Sprained wrists tend to be swollen and sore, with diminished range of motion of the wrist, hand, and even the fingers. Treatment consists of determining the principal distortion types present and applying the proper techniques. A great majority of the time continuum distortions are to blame for wrist sprains, but triggerbands and folding distortions are also relatively common.

Although carpal tunnel syndrome tends to be a long-standing condition that is generally treated in the office setting, some patients will present to the ER to seek a second opinion. The FDM etiology of CTS is either triggerbands or cylinder distortions, with cylinders being more common. To treat the cylinder CTS, locate the area of most discomfort (usually the anterior retinaculum) and place the tip of one thumb lateral and one thumb medial to the distortion. The medial thumb applies firm pressure and pulls the retinaculum medially while at the same time the lateral thumb pulls laterally. Hold in this position as long as possible or until there is a release. Next the thumb position is changed so that one thumb pulls proximally while the other pulls distally. Again force is held until there is a lessening in the tautness of the tissue. In carpal tunnel syndrome it is often beneficial to treat multiple areas of the retinaculum until there is a satisfactory result. Since in CTS the cylinder fascia becomes more and more tangled each time the offending action is repeated, it is generally the result of multiple repetitive behaviors and is best treated in the out-patient setting.

Triggerbands of the wrist are, of course, treated with triggerband technique. The usual locations of these distortions are along the radial and ulnar styloid processes and central posterior wrist. Folding distortions of the wrist can be either unfoldings or refoldings. Unfoldings are treated with a traction/whip technique, while refoldings are corrected with a compression/thrust manipulation.

HAND PAIN

In the hand, continuum distortions outnumber triggerbands as the most common fascial injury seen in the emergency room setting. When working in this very intricate and compact part of the body, the finesse involved in treating is analogous to sculpting — it is an art. The triggerbands are short (as tiny as one-half inch long) and mostly originate and terminate in the hand itself (although some continue onto the fingers). Continuum distortions also are quite small and are palpated under and along the carpal bones. Folding distortions are less common, but when they do occur are also very tiny and delicate. The treatment sequence for hand injuries include:
1. Differentiating the injury into its principal distortion components
2. Correcting them one by one with the appropriate techniques

Generally speaking, in an acute hand injury, triggerbands are treated first, followed by folding distortions, and finally continuum distortions.

THUMB AND FINGER SPRAINS

Sprains of the thumb generally involve continuum distortions in or near the joints and triggerbands of the thenar eminence. Treatment begins by eliciting pain with extension and palpating and correcting the distortions that cause the discomfort. First treat distortions that inhibit extension then treat those affecting flexion. Another injury to the thumb is known by orthopathists as *triggerband thumb*. This is a refolding injury that occurs at the metacarpal-phalangeal joint secondary to performing triggerband technique. The treatment is either refolding technique, or better yet, continuing to treat patients with triggerband technique (this compresses the fascia and allows it to unfold more completely).

Triggerbands in fingers tend to wrap around the digit several times before terminating at the distal tuft; so for an effective treatment the twist must be palpated and corrected along its entire winding course. Stubbed fingers have two etiologies: continuum distortions and refoldings (which are more common). Continuum finger sprains are treated with a very precise continuum technique in which the most distal aspect of the thumb-tip is used to make the correction. Refolding finger sprains are treated with compression/thrust manipulation followed by traction/thrust manipulation.

Cylinder distortions of the finger (symptoms include numbness and tingling) are commonly associated with carpal tunnel syndrome and are treated by applying Indian burn cylinder technique. In this procedure, traction is initiated into the affected portion of the digit with concurrent torquing. The proximal portion of the digit is first rotated in a clockwise direction as the distal portion is rotated in a counterclockwise direction. If the symptoms are unchanged, repeat the procedure with the direction of rotation reversed. And finally, unfolding distortions are also possible in a finger sprain. These are treated with traction/thrust of the affected joint.

NECK PAIN

Most cervical strains seen in the ER are from motor vehicle accidents. In a patient brought in by ambulance on a backboard with a cervical collar in place, the following steps should be considered:
1. Continued immobilization of the neck until it can be properly examined
2. Quick general exam of the entire body to look for other injuries
3. X-rays of cervical spine (if necessary)
4. Providing there are no fractures or other serious injuries, perform physical and structural exam of the neck with documentation of active and passive motion
5. In non-serious injuries, observe body language and correlate with physical findings, verbal description of discomfort, and mechanism of injury to make the orthopathic diagnosis
6. Treat associated fascial distortions one by one
7. Document subjective response, range of motion, and other objective findings before discharge
8. Instruct patient to apply ice if there is pain, and to avoid hot showers and placing heat on the neck for 3-5 days

The treatment of cervical strains is discussed in Chapter 10. However, the emergency room physician should be aware that high-velocity low-amplitude osteopathic manipulation can be safely performed on appropriate patients when the following criteria are met:
- Normal X-ray
- Orthopathic diagnosis is certain
- There are no contraindications (such as fractures, dislocations, severe osteoporosis or rheumatoid arthritis)
- Physician is skilled at performing HVLA

Wry Neck

Wry neck is a special type of acute neck pain in which the sternocleidomastoid muscle spasms. Typical presentation of this condition occurs in patients with no known injury who unexpectedly wake up with pain. Body posture for wry neck patients typically includes head side-bent toward the side of the spasm with the chin rotated away from the spasm. In the orthopathic approach, wry necks are considered to be nothing more than triggerbands of the SCM. Treatment is performed with the patient supine. The neck is gently guided into the position of discomfort with the non-treating hand. The treating thumb then applies firm pressure to the base of the SCM to locate the triggerband. Once found, it is pushed up along the SCM to its termination at the mastoid. After conclusion of triggerband technique, consider thrusting manipulation of the neck, which may reduce residual stiffness by correcting secondary facet tectonic fixations or paravertebral folding distortions. Note that high-velocity thrusting should not be performed until after triggerband technique has been completed. With wry neck triggerbands (and all acute injuries) heat should be avoided both before and after the treatment. Remember the mantra . . . *ice, ice, ice is always nice, nice, nice.*

THORACIC STRAIN

In the acute thoracic strain, just as with any other injury, the mechanism of insult is correlated with the physical findings, description of pain, and body language to determine anatomically which fascial distortions are present. The most common symptoms in acute thoracic strains are pulling or burning pains from the middle upper back to the mastoid. This description of discomfort is pathognomonic for the star triggerband (see Figure 10-1) which is the most commonly encountered triggerband in the body — both in the ER and in the office setting. Treatment is, of course, with triggerband technique from just medial to the mid-scapula up to the mastoid (ipsilateral mastoid 90%, contralateral mastoid 10%). The difference in which route the triggerband takes is dependent on which fascial fibers are injured.

Other common triggerbands include the upper trapezius (which runs from the tip of the shoulder to the mastoid on the same side, see Figure 10-2) and the periscapulars. The periscapular triggerbands tend to have pathways around and under the wing of the scapula. They are generally treated with the patient standing and leaning forward with the elbows bent and the palms chest-high against a wall. The doctor's thumb palpates deep under the scapular wing until the distortion is located, and using triggerband technique *pulls it out* and corrects it along its course to the ipsilateral mastoid. (Note that continuum distortions also occur along the edge of the scapula).

Thoracic continuum distortions tend to occur along the ligaments that connect the transverse processes, and hurt in one or more spots. Treatment is continuum technique with the patient sitting, side-bent, and rotated. This places the patient into the position of injury and allows the treating thumb to get right on top of the distortion. And since most of these continuums are inverted distortions, HVLA in the chair adds to the effect of continuum technique.

Folding distortions of the thoracic paravertebral fascia are quite common and left untreated are a major etiology of so-called chronic back pain. Treatment in the ER consists of the chair technique with either traction or compression — depending on whether the underlying distortion is an unfolding or refolding. Note that unfoldings in the thoracic spine are much more common than refoldings and that the best technique (by far) for the upper thoracic spine is the hallelujah maneuver (see Figure 6-4).

Rib Injuries and Chest Wall Strain

Most sore ribs from a traumatic event can be classified into four categories:
- Strain
- Fracture
- Slipping rib syndrome
- Flail chest

Rib strains are generally comprised of continuum distortions or triggerbands which can be differentiated from each other by the characteristic body languages (continuum = pointing to spot(s) of tenderness or pain, triggerband = sweeping motion of fingers along painful rib). Note that the star folding rib strain is discussed in Chapter 10.

Rib fractures typically present almost identically to that of rib strains, but are distinguished from them by a positive x-ray. However, since the orthopathic treatment is identical for fractures as it is for strains, radiological confirmation does not change the therapeutic course and is therefore considered to be optional (providing there is no suspicion of pneumothorax or other emergent condition).

Treatment of continuum rib strain/fracture:
- Patient seated as thorax is guided into position of maximum discomfort
- Firm pressure is applied with the thumb into the most intense spot(s) of pain and held until release

Treatment of triggerband rib strain/fracture:
- Patient seated as thorax is guided into position of maximum discomfort
- Starting point is appreciated as the most tender portion of pain that pulls along rib
- Thumb is pushed into starting point and forces triggerband twist to move
- Twisted fascial fibers are *ironed out* along entire pathway (generally 3-6")

As you can imagine, both continuum and triggerband techniques for sore ribs are painful. However, it must be remembered how much pain these patients are already in. Some complain of *biting* pain with each breath, and others live in fear of coughing or sneezing. For these people the traditional approach of medicating and waiting weeks for the discomfort to slowly dissipate on its own, is an unacceptable option.

Slipping rib syndrome is a condition in which the lower anterior ribs overlap. Symptoms include a gripping but intermittent pain that is so severe that some patients are forced to sleep in a reclining chair. Treatment: place the patient supine, first refold and then forcefully unfold the intercostal membrane of the overlapping ribs.

Flail chest is a medical emergency in which there is an unstable chest wall due to multiple rib fractures. It is often associated with dyspnea, accelerated respiratory rate, hypoxia, and biting pain with inspiration. Although medical interventions generally involve oxygen, sedation, analgesics, and intubation, some of these responses can be avoided if the level of pain can be functionally reduced. Fortunately, correcting peristernal continuum distortions and triggerbands often substantially lessens the sharp discomfort of inspiration. The reduction in pain allows the patient to take deeper and slower breaths, which decrease the respiratory rate, increase PO2, and diminish the need for intubation.

In contrast to flail chest is simple chest wall strain, which results from a single activity such as swinging a baseball bat. These injuries are again broken down into their fascial distortion components (triggerbands and continuums are most common) and treated with the appropriate fascial distortion technique.

KIDNEY STONE PAIN

Renal colic pain is commonly encountered in the Emergency Department. The traditional therapeutic and diagnostic approaches generally include hydration with intravenous fluids, narcotic analgesics, and IVP studies. Although these methods have merit, most patients with renal colic continue to have substantial pain (which is often intolerable) for hours on end.

In the fascial distortion model, renal calculi are viewed as a normal occurrence. Everyone, or at least many people, routinely pass kidney stones. Few, however, suffer from renal colic. What separates asymptomatic people from those who experience discomfort is a fascial distortion constricting the ureter and keeping the stone from passing. Clinically there are two types of fascial distortions which result in renal colic: herniated triggerpoints and triggerbands. Both are found in the flank, with herniated triggerpoints being the more common of the two. These patients complain of a dull ache in their side and present to the Emergency Department with an unmistakable body language — their thumb pushing into the herniated triggerpoint. On physical exam, palpation of the HTP reproduces and magnifies the pain. The body language of triggerband renal colic patients, in contrast, consists of a sweeping motion from the flank to the groin.

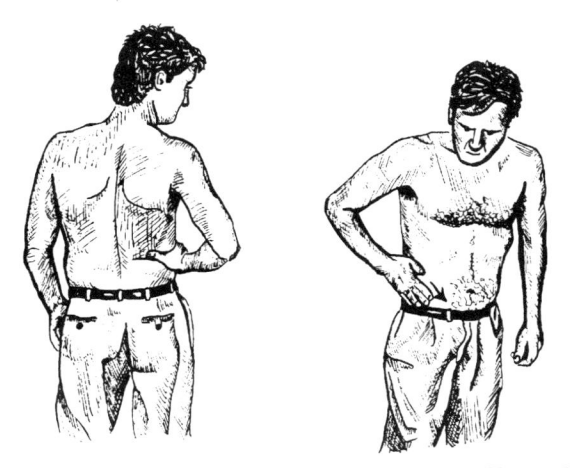

Figure 13-1. Body Language of Flank HTP (left) and Flank Triggerband (right)

Treatment of the *flank HTP* consists of herniated triggerpoint therapy (i.e., pushing into the pain with the tip of the thumb and holding force until resolution). The amount of force necessary for correction is substantial — so much so that the doctor may need to use his/her knee to help push the elbow (and thereby the thumb) into the flank HTP. When resolution of the flank herniated triggerpoint occurs, there is either a dramatic reduction in pain or the pain is completely eliminated. Note that the release itself is perhaps the largest of any herniated triggerpoint in the body and is easily appreciated by both physician and patient.

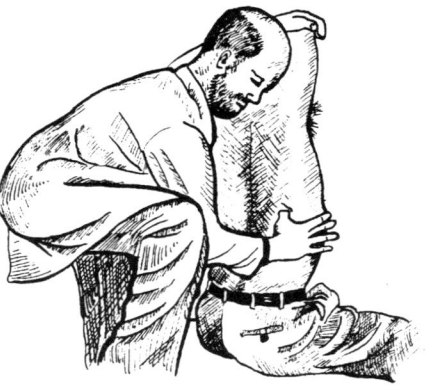

Figure 13-2. Treatment of Flank HTP

Triggerband renal colic is obviously treated with triggerband technique. These patients complain of pain in the flank that radiates into the abdomen or groin. To treat, the thumb first locates the distortion deep in the flank and then irons it out along its entire pathway through the abdomen to the groin.

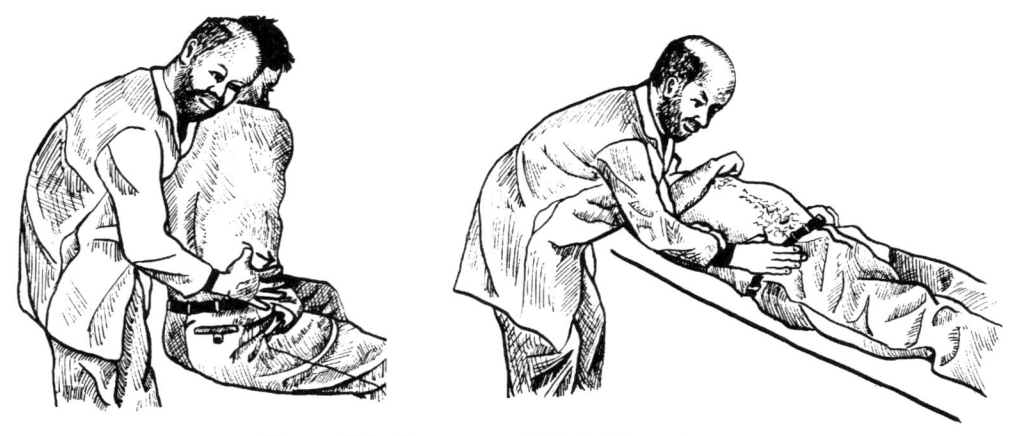

Figure 13-3. Treatment of Flank Triggerband

Following a successful treatment with either technique, the patient should be observed in the ER for an hour or so to be sure that there is no reoccurrence of pain. If there is, the treatment should be repeated. Typically, about half the patients with severe renal colic pain who are treated with FDM techniques will leave the ER pain-free without having needed IV narcotics or even a prescription. Of those who respond, most do so within only 60 seconds after initiating the procedure. Some patients even feel the stone pass during the treatment.

Those patients who don't get complete relief will still report some subjective benefit from the therapy. A reduction in discomfort from a ten on arrival to a four after the treatment is typical (on a scale of 0-10). Small doses of narcotic medicine can then be given to further decrease pain. Surprisingly, most patients who only moments before were adamantly requesting medication, and who obtained only partial relief of pain with the FDM treatment, will then refuse all analgesic medications.

GALL BLADDER ATTACKS

Acute biliary pain from a gallstone in the bile duct may respond to fascial distortion techniques. In the FDM, gall bladder attacks have a similar mechanism to that of renal colic (i.e., the bile duct is being partially constricted by a fascial distortion). When the distortion is corrected, the stone passes, alleviating the pain. Clinically, biliary colic presents as several herniated triggerpoints in the region of the gall bladder. They are particularly tender to the touch but otherwise behave much the same as other types of HTP's. Gall bladder HTP's are treated by holding firm pressure with the thumb directly into the distortion until it completely releases. The time it takes before the release begins is variable, depending upon how easily the thumb is able to focus directly into the distortion. Again it may be helpful to milk the HTP during its release (this eases the tissue back below the fascial plane).

Some biliary colic patients present with triggerbands rather than herniated triggerpoints. These patients are treated by first palpating the distortion near the gall bladder and then *pulling the triggerband out into the abdomen*. From there it is corrected along its course to the xyphoid process where the pathway terminates. Note that fascial distortion treatments are not designed to be a substitute for medical and/or surgical assessment. Instead they are intended to reduce or eliminate the pain, which is of primary concern to the patient.

ABDOMINAL AND PELVIC PAIN

Fascial distortion techniques in the abdomen consist of herniated triggerpoint therapy and triggerband technique. These two modalities can at times be quite helpful for eliminating or reducing pain from a wide variety of ailments such as painful ovulation and pancreatitis (see Case History #23). Caution must be exercised when interpreting the results of abdominal FDM therapies because the success of the treatments may mask the seriousness of an acute surgical situation. So before FDM treatments are initiated, the medical ramifications of the therapy must be contemplated.

In acute abdominal pain, herniated triggerpoints are generally treated before triggerbands (if they are present). For some, one HTP will be the sole cause of pain; while in other cases, three or four may exist. In chronic abdominal pain, dozens of HTP's and triggerbands are expected. The treatment of abdominal HTP's includes applying firm pressure deep into the abdomen and palpating the distortion. Be sure that the discomfort is maximized and that the treating thumb has the proper direction of force. Hold the HTP firmly and milk it as it releases.

Abdominal triggerbands are located in the same fashion as abdominal HTP's, that is with the tip of the thumb. In the abdomen, the thumb must *worm* its way through the layers of tissue until the distortion is palpated. Then the triggerband is pushed into the direction that increases the pain. In this manner, the triggerband is *dug out* of the abdomen and forced either to the sternum or to the pelvis where the fibers terminate. When treating abdominal pain, it is advisable to keep patients in the ER at least one hour following the treatment to be sure that their pain does not reoccur. If it does, then re-evaluate and consider re-treating. Note that soreness and bruising from the treatment are not uncommon.

LOW BACK PAIN

Patients with acute lumbar sprains commonly show up in the Emergency Room late at night (and often by ambulance) when they are in excruciating pain. The primary reason that this occurs so frequently is that they have been instructed to "put heat on it." The obliging patients generally do so in the following fashion:
1. During the early evening a hot shower is taken. Initially the back feels better, but . . . some three hours later, he/she experiences increasing pain, so . . .
2. Another hot shower is taken, this time with only half the relief. Three hours later, the pain has intensified, so . . .
3. One more hot shower is taken
4. Several hours following hot shower #3 the patient is in so much pain he or she calls for an ambulance

The first clinical response by the ER doctor should be to treat with an *ice massage* (not an ice pack). The ice should be directly applied to the skin and kept in slow, constant motion. (Don't be distracted by the worry of frostbite.) Secondly, the patient should be instructed not to take any hot showers or baths and reminded to apply ice.

Next the patient is evaluated medically, orthopedically, and orthopathically. Fortunately, many of the low back pain cases will have one or more of the following personalities which can be treated with fascial distortion techniques (see Chapter 10):
- *Pain over sacroiliac joint that pulls down posterior thigh* – treat with triggerband technique along the low back pain with thigh tightness triggerband
- *Pulling or burning pain down lateral thigh* – treat with triggerband technique along the iliotibial band
- *Pain in gluteal bull's-eye* – treat with herniated triggerpoint therapy
- *Pain in one spot over sacroiliac joint* – treat with continuum technique (these are inverted distortions) followed by thrusting manipulation (scissors technique)
- *Pain deep in lumbar spine* – treat with chair folding technique
- *Squeezing pain across entire lower portion of low back* – treat with double thumb cylinder technique
- *Pain deep at base of lumbar spine* – treat with frogleg and reverse frogleg tectonic techniques of hip

GROIN STRAIN

Pulled groin muscles in the fascial distortion model are treated as triggerbands. Treatment consists of finding the origin of the triggerband in the thigh and following it into the groin with triggerband technique. If the patient continues to complain of pain or says that the pain has moved, this means that either inadequate force was applied or the triggerband was not completely re-zipped.

THIGH PAIN

Perhaps the two most common presentations of fascial thigh pain are hamstring pulls and quadriceps strains. Both of these are typically treated as triggerbands. Hamstring pulls involve a triggerband in the posterior muscles of the thigh. The distorted band is palpated as a large and tender *knot* (triggerband subtype). To treat, a good deal of force is needed to *drag* the triggerband through the belly of the muscle. This particular distortion elicits the *burning* sensation for which triggerband technique is so well known. The hamstring pathway begins as a triggerband knot, then runs deep into and through the involved muscle to the plane below. Once the triggerband is pushed through the muscle, the treatment is complete. Ice massage and re-treatment in 24 hours are advised. Quadriceps strains are very similar to hamstring pulls but they occur on the anterior aspect of the thigh. Treatment consists of first locating the triggerband knot and pushing it deep into and through the involved muscle. Note that both quadriceps strains and hamstring pulls involve triggerband treatments in three dimensions (i.e., the direction of force is straight through the muscle).

Patients with cylinder distortions of the thigh rarely present to the Emergency Department since their symptoms tend to be generalized and less severe than hamstring or quadriceps pulls. Most describe the discomfort as a deep ache in the center of the thigh. Treatment is with Indian burn cylinder technique in which traction and torque are used. Because of the size of the thigh, this is perhaps the most difficult cylinder treatment of all. For some patients, it may be necessary to first treat the anterior aspect, then the medial, then the posterior, and finally the lateral. In this way, the thigh is circled like a clock. Other options include squeegee technique and double thumb compression cylinder variant (see Figure 7-7).

KNEE SPRAINS

Knee sprains may have what appear to be many different orthopedic presentations, but most can be readily divided into their fascial distortion types. Continuum distortions and triggerbands are commonly palpated on the anterior medial aspect of the knee along the tibio-femoral joint. Following a twisting injury to the knee, a continuum distortion or triggerband may form in this space. Often these patients can't fully flex or extend the knee and there may be a significant amount of swelling. To treat, firmly palpate the distortion with your thumb. If it moves, treat it as a triggerband. If it doesn't move, then treat it as a continuum distortion (i.e., apply strong pressure directly into the space and hold until release). During treatment, triggerband distortions of the anterior medial knee move up and out of the joint and onto the anterior thigh. Continuum distortions, which are more common, may occur singly or in pairs.

Another common knee distortion involves the distal thigh just above the patella. In these knee sprains there is typically swelling and loss of flexion. The distortion is located by palpating the area and applying firm pressure. If it can be induced to move, it is a triggerband. Treat by pushing it superiorly toward the thigh. In acute knee sprains this pathway is normally only two or three inches long. If the distortion is a continuum distortion, it will reside deeper in the tissue and will be on top of the bone. To treat, hold it firmly and precisely until it releases.

Cylinder distortions of the knee are rarely seen in the ER setting. Most patients feel that since the pain is diffuse and there is little or no swelling, the injury is of a less serious nature. Treatment of cylinder knee sprains is generally with Indian burn cylinder technique.

Unfolding knee sprains result from the joint being hyperextended, such as occurs from missing a step on a stairway. Treatment consists of traction or traction/thrust in which the knee is tugged on in a number of different directions. When the treatment is successful a small or large pop will be heard. Refolding knee sprains are less common and develop from jamming the knee. The pain is similar to an unfolding in that they both hurt deep in the joint. The difference clinically is that unfolding knee sprains hurt with compression and feel better with traction, whereas refolding knee sprains hurt if they are tractioned and feel better if they are compressed. The treatment of refoldings is therefore with compression/thrust. The most effective refolding manipulation of the knee is with the patient supine and the joint bent at a 60° angle. The physician cradles the heel with his or her interlaced hands and thrusts the foot superiorly towards the knee which is stabilized against the treating chest.

LEG PAIN

Shin splints come in two varieties: triggerbands and continuum distortions (triggerbands are more common). The two are differentiated by the patient's description of pain and body language. Triggerbands pull up (or down) the leg while continuum distortions hurt in specific spots. Frequently patients will use a sweeping motion with their hand to show a triggerband, but with a continuum distortion they will point with one finger. Triggerband shin splints occur along the medial or lateral border of the tibia with the entire pathway contained within the leg itself. Treatment consists of finding the triggerband and correcting it along its course. Note that shin splint triggerbands are commonly abutted against the tibia. Continuum shin splints rarely occur alone, but often are found in pairs or trios. As with other continuum distortions, treatment consists of guiding the leg into the position of most pain, applying direct pressure with the treating thumb into the distortion, and holding until it releases.

In the distal leg, folding distortions occur within the interosseous membrane and are particularly common following ankle and leg fractures. In the ER, a gentle traction force may help separate the tibia and fibula and correct the unfolding injury. Refolding distortions rarely occur in fractures but are common in post-stroke spastic paralysis patients. These injuries are treated with a strong thrust so that the two hands compress the tibia and fibula together. A pop or loud crack signifies that the correction has been made.

Cylinder leg distortions are most common in the elderly. These patients exhibit a typical *cylinder shuffle* gait as they walk which is reminiscent of the *P.I.D. shuffle* that women get with uterine infections. Leg cylinder distortions are more than just a nuisance. If left uncorrected, edema and cellulitis can develop along with unrelenting discomfort. Unfortunately many of these older folks become frustrated with conventional treatments and end up being permanently wheelchair-bound. Treatment consists of squeegee technique (see Figure 7-6), double thumb cylinder technique, or Indian burn cylinder technique.

ANKLE SPRAINS

Acute ankle sprains occur in three varieties: continuum, triggerband, and folding. Continuum sprained ankles are the most common and typically occur from a sudden eversion injury (i.e., the ankle buckles outward). Triggerband ankle sprains result from the leg becoming twisted, which torques the fascial fibers and ligaments causing triggerbands. The third and least common ankle sprain is the folding type. These sprained ankles result when something (or somebody) is holding the foot down at the time of mishap.

Although at first glance all three ankle sprains look alike (i.e., they're swollen, weak, and tender), the anatomical distortions are different and thus the treatment approaches also are different. Continuum sprained ankles are treated with continuum technique, triggerband sprained ankles with triggerband technique, and folding sprained ankles with folding technique. Note that refolding ankle sprains tend to have mild symptoms so few of these patients initially present at the Emergency Room, but instead tend to wait for the ankle to "heal on its own." Acute ankle sprains and their treatments are discussed in more detail in Chapter 12.

FOOT SPRAINS

Foot sprains may consist of triggerbands, continuum distortions, folding distortions, or cylinder distortions. Triggerbands in the foot generally are treated from proximal to distal, and terminate at the end of one of the toes. Continuum distortions may be of either the everted or inverted type and both are treated with continuum technique.

Patients with a folding sprained foot typically exhibit swelling and complain of pain deep between the bones. In unfolding treatments, both hands are used to pull the metatarsal bones gently apart. This allows the folding fascia to unfold and then refold uncontorted.

Refolding distortions occur if the foot is squeezed, and treatment consists of compressing the foot and allowing the fascia to subsequently unfold.

Cylinder distortions give a vague sensation of deep pain in the foot. Treatment consists of the double thumb method in which first the deeper layer is treated and then the more superficial layer. The deeper layer is corrected by having one thumb maintain traction in a medial direction while the other thumb does so in a lateral direction. The superficial layer is then corrected by having the proximal thumb pull proximally while the distal thumb pulls distally. In either case, traction is held until the tissue tautness diminishes.

PLANTAR FASCIITIS

Pain from plantar fasciitis is encountered much more frequently in the office setting than the ER. Clinically, it presents as a diffuse tightness along the entire length of the bottom of the foot. In addition, there is typically a small point of excruciating tenderness along the plantar edge of the calcaneus. The complaint of tightness originates from a triggerband that extends from the calcaneus to the base of the toes and the small spot of pain is secondary to a continuum distortion at the origin of the plantar fascia on the calcaneus. Note that if a bone spur has formed, this is evidence that the distortion is pulling bony products into the fascia.

The strategy of treatment is first to correct the triggerband and then to treat the continuum distortion. Treatment of either requires great thumb strength and stamina. Triggerbands are treated along the plantar fascia from the calcaneus to the metatarsal-phalangeal junction. The continuum distortion is palpated deep in the tissue at the edge of the calcaneus and to successfully correct this *heel spur continuum distortion* requires more strength and skill than perhaps any other in the entire body. To treat, the thumb is wormed through the thick plantar fascia until the distortion is located and then pressure from the very tip is focused and held until the release. Since this particular problem is a constant annoyance, most patients are enthusiastically appreciative of the physician's efforts.

TOE SPRAINS AND FRACTURES

Although several different fascial distortion types can present in the fractured or sprained toe, the most common are continuum distortions. They occur at the fracture site (or in sprains at the origin or insertion of the toe ligament or tendon). Despite their small size, they are fairly easy to palpate and correct using continuum technique. To treat, firm pressure is applied to the most tender spot and held until release. Although the fracture is still visible on x-ray, a successful treatment results in the patient being able to wear a shoe and walk without pain.

Chapter 14

THE ORTHOPATHIC APPROACH TO TREATING POST-STROKE SPASTIC PARALYSIS

In the fascial distortion model, the spastic paralysis of an extremity that so often follows a stroke is considered to be the cumulative result of:

1. *Uncorrected fascial distortions that anatomically restrict movement* – Multitudes of distortions form during the initial flaccid paralytic period when muscle tone is diminished secondary to a temporary loss of neurological input. Without the support of the partially contracting muscle fibers, the fascia within and around affected muscles physically crumple upon themselves. Once neurological input returns, these distortions anatomically inhibit muscle contractions (both active and passive), resulting in *stiffness*.

2. *Scrambling of electrical impulses through the distorted fascial network* diffuses neuro input to the target muscle (i.e., the muscle that the brain is commanding to move). Once the flaccid period is over, electrical impulses originating in the brain flood into the paralyzed areas, but because of the altered fascia, only a small portion of them are properly distributed within the target muscle. These deficient muscular contractions are interpreted by patients as *weakness*.

3. *Spilling out of electrical impulses from the target muscle into adjacent flexors and extensors* – The intermuscular septa and interosseous membranes when contorted are unable to isolate and buffer neighboring muscle groups from the electrical impulses passing into the target muscle. This spill-over causes *hypertonicity*, *spasm*, and *tremors*, since at any given time, commanding one muscle to contract results in other muscles also contracting.

The spastic or reflex-like movements so typical of post-stroke patients are, from an orthopathic perspective, considered not to be involuntary and purposeless, but instead voluntary yet spastic. In the FDM any muscle movement of any kind (even spasm, tremor, or hypertonia) is considered to be triggered by signals from the brain commanding that muscle to move. In the post-stroke patient, this tends to occur in an uncoordinated fashion. The resultant movement is therefore voluntary. But since the signal spills over into adjacent muscle groups, the desired movement of individual muscles cannot be isolated and is instead accompanied by tremor (alternating spilling of electricity back and forth from flexors to extensors), spasm (simultaneous but intermittent stimulation of both flexors and extensors), or hypertonicity (continuous stimulation of the involved muscle groups).

The primary goal in the orthopathic treatment of post-stroke spastic paralysis is to *change muscular movements from voluntary/spastic to voluntary/controlled*. This is done in the following manner:

I. *Eliminate fascial distortions.*

II. *Consciously link together isolated spastic motions with seemingly unrelated coordinated motions.* For instance, flexing of the non-paralyzed right knee may initiate extension of the paralyzed left third finger. The patient is encouraged to mentally link these two behaviors together, so that when asked to extend the left third finger this can be done by first flexing the right knee.

III. *Mentally extinguish associated non-spastic motions so that when the brain commands movement only the spastic motion remains.* In the above example the patient is taught to concentrate on extending the finger but to mentally inhibit flexion of the knee. In a short time, the finger extends without the knee flexing — thus making this motion both voluntary and coordinated.

IV. *Mentally extinguish other undesirable movements or behaviors.* Commonly in post-stroke patients with hemiplegia, movement of a spastic muscle elicits other seemingly unrelated spastic motions. In the case of the paralyzed left third finger, extension is often accompanied with unwanted flexion of the same-side elbow. The unsolicited elbow flexion is extinguished by first correcting associated regional fascial distortions (particularly cylinder and folding distortions of the elbow and forearm), and then by mentally inhibiting elbow flexion when practicing third finger extension.

It should be noted that some post-stroke spastic paralysis patients (PSSPP) mentally exhaust themselves attempting to move their spastic limbs. Unfortunately, since the excess electrical impulses generated by their brains simply spill over into the adjacent muscle groups, the result is amplification of muscle tone, spasm, and tremor. Instead of *trying hard*, these individuals should be encouraged to *think gently*, and reminded that it doesn't take much strength to move a finger!

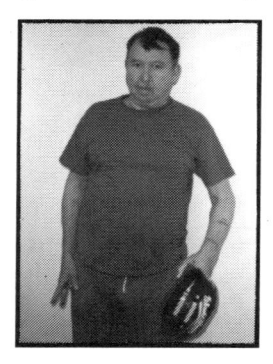

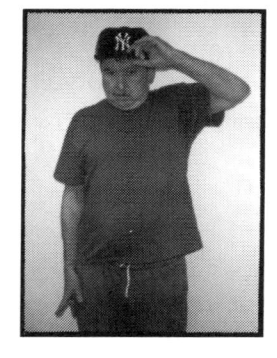

Figure 14-1. Patient with left upper extremity post-stroke spastic paralysis shown putting cap on for first time since stroke
CVA – thirteen months ago
Shoulder motion prior to FDM treatments – abduction and flexion both 70°
Number of orthopathic treatments – 4

Philosophy of Treatment

STEP I: Correct Fascial Distortions

The fascial distortions that form during a stroke not only scramble and diffuse electrical stimulation, but also physically restrict movement. This straitjacket effect keeps the target muscle from adequately contracting and triggers the positive feedback loop of the nervous system to repeat the command with increased electrical volume. However, the excess electricity is counter-productive since it spills into and stimulates neighboring muscles, thereby creating for the PSSPP a *spastic merry-go-round* — the more he or she tries to move, the more spasm results.

The restrictions of large conglomerations of fascial injuries can be clinically lumped together into general terms such as those listed below:

Frozen shoulder	Frozen hip
Frozen elbow	Frozen knee
Frozen wrist	Frozen ankle

In orthopathy, the initial approach in treating the PSSPP is essentially the same as has been discussed in other sections of the book: Break the gross restrictions down into their components and treat them with fascial distortion techniques. For instance, in a typical treatment scenario for the frozen shoulder component of the stroke, the shoulder is examined and treated as discussed in Chapter 11. Virtually all of these patients have a chronic sore shoulder with global loss of active and passive range of motion (see Orthopathic Flow Chart of the Chronically Sore Shoulder). The treatment begins with the SCHTP and triggerband technique (the star, upper trapezius, and anterior and posterior shoulder pathways, and possibly the comb technique). Following several days of rest the shoulder is re-treated. If there is still global loss of passive motion, slow tectonic pump and tectonic technique (frogleg and reverse frogleg) are employed. It may be helpful to apply wet heat and use the plunger technique before the manipulation. If the motion remains unimproved, repeat the sequence several times in the next two weeks and consider prone tectonic technique (see glossary term *Prone Tectonic Technique of the Shoulder*).

Once the shoulder has some improved passive range of motion, it now has the possibility of acquiring at least some active motion. However, folding distortions in the interosseous membrane of the forearm and tectonic fixations of the wrist and elbow still limit motion. These are corrected with a modified frogleg for the elbow, thrusting manipulation of the flexed wrist, and traction/thrust or compression/thrust manipulation of the forearm.

As the shoulder, wrist, and forearm become passively looser, attention is then directed to the hand which generally presents as a perpetually clenched fist. Folding distortions of the interosseous membranes are particularly responsible for this and are treated with folding/thrusting manipulation of the membranes surrounding the lumbricals.

Frozen hips of PSSPP's are treated with triggerband technique (the lateral thigh and posterior thigh pathways) and then frogleg and reverse frogleg techniques. Folding distortions also are common and may inhibit tectonic technique. If the hip is placed into the frogleg position and pain is elicited deep in the joint, this means that an unfolding distortion of the hip is present. When there are concurrent folding distortions and tectonic fixations of the hip, the folding distortion must be corrected first (this is because tectonic technique causes the fascia to fold into an even more contorted configuration). Be aware that a successful folding treatment of the hip requires a large amount of traction or compression plus physician strength.

Once the folding distortion is corrected (evident by the frogleg position no longer being painful), tectonic technique is performed. Please note that the direction and positioning of frogleg and reverse frogleg can be modified to engage either the knee or the ankle. In either case, tectonic fixations of these two areas can be treated at the same time.

Fascial Distortions and Loss of Sensation

Many PSSPP's complain of patches or large areas of numbness in the paralyzed extremity or trunk. This loss of sensation is thought to occur in part because of fascial distortions blocking mechanical fascial sensory information to the nervous system. Triggerbands and cylinder distortions are the most common distortions involved, and treatment of them may subjectively improve sensation.

Iliotibial Tract Triggerbands and Balance

The correction of triggerbands of the iliotibial band is a major component in improving proprioception and balance. The results of these treatments are typically immediate and can be documented with a stopwatch. To do so, have the patient stand on one foot and measure the time he or she can balance, then repeat the process on the other foot. Following treatment, measure the difference.

STEP II: Link Together Spastic Motions with Coordinated Motions

As Step I progresses, spasm decreases and passive range of motion increases. The stroke victim is obviously more comfortable — but still paralyzed. However, even in this semi-flaccid state the patient may suddenly spasm. If, for instance, he or she is sitting comfortably, and an attempt is made to move an uninjured portion of the body this may cause the paralyzed arm or leg to move. By isolating the exact movement that triggers the spastic movement we can teach the patient to consciously reproduce the sequence. In this manner, for example, flexing the opposite non-paralyzed hip is followed by flexion of the paralyzed shoulder. In just a few minutes some patients can grasp this concept and learn to control the pattern so that when commanded by the doctor to flex the paralyzed shoulder this can be accomplished by first flexing the non-paralyzed hip.

This step regains gross yet voluntary movement. The more links that can be made between the non-paralyzed movements and the paralyzed limb, the more overall movements can be regained. In a sense, Step II reprograms the neuro pathway for motion to the paralyzed limb by using a more accessible trigger mechanism somewhere else in the body.

STEP III: Stop the Triggering Movement

In Step II we are able to regain new motion through secondary triggering mechanisms. However, it is highly undesirable to have to physically perform one action (flex a hip) to get another (flex the opposite shoulder). So in Step III the patient consciously thinks of the triggering mechanism but at the same time inhibits the actual activation of it. Generally, within only a few sessions the spastic motion can be commanded without having to physically employ the triggering movement. Surprisingly, the activation of the new motion becomes unconsciously ingrained to such an extent that it remains easily accessible even after the triggering mechanism is consciously long forgotten.

STEP IV: Stop Other Unnecessary Movements

Although in Step III the triggering movement is extinguished, other unnecessary movements may still exist. For instance, when the command is given to flex the wrist, excess electricity spills out into neighboring muscle groups causing the elbow to flex and the wrist to pronate. These accessory and undesirable movements greatly diminish the usefulness of the motion and are an endless source of frustration for the patient.

The spilling of electricity into adjacent muscle groups occurs because of one or more of the following three mechanisms:
1. Scrambling of neurological input
2. Unconsciously commanding other muscles to contract
3. Amount of electricity is far in excess of what is required to cause the desired movement

Extinguishing the accessory movements occurs by:
1. Correcting regionally associated fascial distortions
2. Mentally focusing only on the desired motion
3. Cutting down the amount of electricity to the muscle(s) that are being commanded to move

So in a PSSPP who demonstrates involuntary movement of the elbow with wrist flexion, the first plan of treatment is to identify and correct any residual fascial distortions. In particular, look for folding distortions of the forearm interosseous membrane (the correction of this difficult injury is with a traction/thrust or compression/thrust procedure), and tectonic fixations of the elbow (treat with a modified frogleg or reverse frogleg technique).

And finally it should be realized that in addition to making physical changes it is also necessary to make mental changes. PSSPP's unwittingly flood the entire paralyzed limb with the mental command of movement, which causes every muscle in the entire extremity to contract. To rectify this *spastic flooding*, patients must mentally focus on the desired movement only and refrain from drawing in help from other portions of the spastic limb.

The third point listed above — cutting down the neurological input — cannot be stressed enough. PSSPP's typically *try too hard* to move the spastic extremity. To combat this tendency they must learn to *think gently*, meaning practicing over and over again moving the paralyzed limb with far less mental command than they feel will ever elicit a response.

A LOOK AHEAD

In the future not only are the treatments for post-stroke spastic paralysis expected to improve markedly, but spastic paralysis itself may be avoided. By correcting fascial distortions as early as possible following the stroke, patients may progress from flaccid paralysis to recovery without passing through the spastic phase.

Section Three

Case Histories

Case History #1 Ankle Pain in a 41 Year Old Man

Chief Complaint: Right ankle pain x 31 years

History: Stepped in hole, twisted foot, and sustained a fracture to his ankle in 1967 (no documentation available about the type or severity of fracture)

Treatments: Casting
Surgery x 1 in 1978 with no change in symptoms
Multiple injections which "helped for a couple of days"

Physicians seen: "Dozens"

Symptoms:
Daily bi-malleolar swelling (worse in afternoon, or after walking, or standing on concrete floors)
Aching deep in ankle
Stiffness of foot (worse in A.M.)
Inability to place foot flat on floor
Walking barefoot increases symptoms
Increase in swelling and pain with even small excursions over irregular ground
Tires easily and has to rest frequently if walking on sandy beach

Physical Exam: Decreased dorsiflexion
Mild bi-malleolar swelling
Small surgical scar present
Decreased and painful active and passive range of motion

X-ray Interpretation: Normal foot and ankle

Orthopedic Impression: Chronic ankle pain

Course of Treatment: Mr. S. was treated orthopathically. At the conclusion of the initial visit he demonstrated improved inversion and eversion and while standing was able to pivot better on the ankle. After the second treatment he stated that he could now stand with the foot feeling as if it were flat on the floor. After the third session he walked for several miles at Sand Beach and the ankle and foot felt "great." Following the fourth treatment he had no more swelling, no symptoms, and he felt as if his foot and ankle were "almost normal again."

Discussion Topic: Orthopathic diagnosis

Case History #1

Orthopathic Diagnosis:
1. Long-standing acute ankle sprain of the folding type
2. Tectonic fixations of the foot

Discussion: Folding distortions of the interosseous membrane are expected with a fracture of the ankle and typically present with the clinical findings of:

1. Aching deep in joint
2. Bi-malleolar swelling
3. Loss of motion

Unfortunately for Mr. S., the folding distortion of the distal tibiofibular interosseous membrane was held in place by the application of a cast which limited the movement, i.e., unfolding and refolding of the membrane. With this limited motion, synovial fluid circulation was decreased and tectonic fixations of the ankle and foot joints formed.

The folding distortions also physically limited the shock-absorbing function of the periarticular fascia which caused the aching discomfort deep in the joint and the aggravation of symptoms when Mr. S. tried to walk on a soft or irregular surface. Note that the correction of the folding distortion facilitated the re-absorption of interstitial swelling by restoring the fascial fluid transport network.

Although children tend to recover more completely than adults from fractures (secondary to the fascia's ability to anatomically minimize the shortening effect of the contorted tissue by lengthening the fascia through growing) this was not the case in Mr. S.'s injury. In this instance the placing of the cast created the tectonic fixations, which then cemented the ankle and leg folding distortions firmly in place and caused the stiffness of the foot.

Since the injury contained none of the body language or physical findings suggestive of triggerbands with adhesions, the injury was considered to be a non-resolved acute sprain rather than a chronic condition. The rapid clinical response to the treatments is also typical of an acute injury.

Case History #2 Shoulder Pain in a 50 Year Old Woman

Chief Complaint: Left shoulder pain x 2 days

History: This pharmaceutical representative injured her left shoulder stocking a shelf with drug samples. As the arm stretched upwards and backwards, Ms. F. felt an excruciating pain deep in the shoulder. Over the next several hours a severe new pain developed in the upper arm along with loss of shoulder motion.

Symptoms: Severe pain deep in shoulder
Severe pain deep in upper arm
Weakness
Loss of motion

Physical Exam:
Abduction   R = 180°   L = 90°
External rotation   R = 90°   L = 60° (slow)
Internal rotation   R = 12" above waist line   L = 3" below waist line
No point tenderness, no palpable fracture
Body language: squeezes upper arm repetitively

X-ray: Not done

Orthopedic Diagnosis: Acutely frozen shoulder

Discussion Topic: Orthopathic diagnosis and treatment

Case History #2
Orthopathic Diagnosis: Acutely frozen shoulder secondary to folding and cylinder distortions

Discussion: Ms. F. sustained an injury that resulted in global loss of motion (i.e., loss of abduction, external, and internal rotation). On the Orthopathic Flow Chart of the Acutely Sore Shoulder there are four possibilities listed: fracture, dislocation, separated shoulder, and cylinder distortion. Taking these one by one:

1. Fracture is unlikely because:
    No point tenderness
    No swelling
    No deformity
    No open wound
    No audible crack
    Mechanism of injury
    Global loss of motion was not immediate

2. Dislocation is unlikely because:
    No palpable dislocation
    Doesn't explain pain in upper arm
    Global loss of motion was not immediate

3. Separated shoulder is unlikely because:
    Pain is not over the acromioclavicular joint
    Mechanism of injury
    Global loss of motion was not immediate

4. Cylinder distortion is likely because:
    Severe pain in upper arm
    Mechanism of injury
    Delay in global loss of motion is typical of cylinder injury

Although in this instance a cylinder distortion is overwhelmingly the most likely culprit for the manifestation of global loss of motion, if there is any concern, an x-ray should be taken to rule out a fracture, dislocation, or separated shoulder. And although a cylinder distortion of the upper arm is clinically consistent with global loss of motion, pain in the upper arm, and body language of repetitively squeezing the biceps or triceps muscle — the diagnosis does not explain the pain deep in the shoulder joint. From an orthopathic perspective, the contorted periarticular folding fascia developed first, and then unequally pulled on the superficial circular fascia and tangled it.

In this case Ms. F. was treated first by unfolding technique (i.e., placing the shoulder into the exact position of injury and reproducing the forces that caused the injury) and then by cylinder technique of the upper arm. She did well on the first treatment with restoration of abduction and external rotation. However, two more visits were required to completely restore internal rotation.

Case History #3 Low Back Pain in a 46 Year Old Man

Mr. W. is a gentleman with a 30 year history of low back pain. Although his low back had been constantly stiff and achy for the entire 30 years, his primary complaint is a pulling pain down his left posterior thigh which developed ten years ago. Mr. W. has no specific recollection of an injury or event that preceded his pain. He has had a long workup which included MRI and other studies (all normal) and has received every available treatment including manipulation, injections, physical therapy, medications, and pain management – all without relief. Mr. W. has been working with pain, gets out of a chair slowly, and stands with a definite curvature to the left. While describing his discomfort it is noted that he is unable to stand fully erect, makes a sweeping motion with his hand inferiorly down the left posterior thigh, then grips the iliac crest with both hands, followed by placing the back of his hand against the lumbar vertebrae.

Discussion Questions:
1. From the description of his symptoms it is likely that Mr. W. has been suffering from:
   A. Gluteal bull's-eye herniated triggerpoint, a tectonic fixation of the hip, and a cylinder distortion of the low back
   B. Lateral thigh tightness triggerband, a folding distortion of the low back, and a continuum distortion of the sacroiliac joint
   C. Folding distortion of the low back and a tectonic fixation of the hip
   D. Folding distortion of the low back, a posterior thigh tightness triggerband, and a tectonic fixation of the hip
   E. Folding distortion of the low back, continuum distortion of the sacroiliac joint (inverted), and a posterior thigh tightness triggerband

2. The first treatment to be employed should be:
   A. Triggerband technique
   B. Herniated triggerpoint therapy
   C. Continuum technique
   D. Cylinder technique
   E. Folding technique
   F. Tectonic technique

3. If folding technique is utilized, the most reasonable first choice would be:
   A. Inversion therapy (ball technique)
   B. Inversion therapy (inversion table)
   C. Traction
   D. Wall technique
   E. Chair technique

4. If tectonic technique is applied, the most reasonable first choice would be:
   A. Slow tectonic pump
   B. Plunger technique
   C. Kirksville crunch
   D. Whip technique
   E. Frogleg and reverse frogleg technique

5. In this particular case the final diagnosis of *chronic low back pain – resolved* was made on the sixth office visit and the patient was discharged. Recheck in four months found him to be pain free and asymptomatic. The reason that his final diagnosis included the term *chronic* was because of the:
   A. Tectonic fixations and triggerbands
   B. Folding distortions and triggerbands
   C. Triggerbands with adhesions
   D. Gluteal bull's-eye HTP
   E. Large length of time of symptoms (30 years)

6. When did Mr. W.'s injury actually become *chronic*?
   A. 30 years ago when the symptoms first occurred
   B. Gradually over a long period of time but impossible to know for sure
   C. The day the diagnosis of chronic low back pain was made
   D. 10 years ago

7. If we were to speculate on how Mr. W.'s back was originally injured, we would guess:
   A. He bent forward and twisted his low back picking up a heavy object in his job as a construction worker
   B. His left foot became caught and he jerked it free
   C. He fell down hard on a concrete floor landing predominantly on his left lower extremity
   D. It was a series of repetitious small injuries (overuse syndrome)

Case History #3
Discussion Questions:

Question #1. Answer: D
  Mr. W.'s body language is clear:
- Places back of hand against lumbar vertebrae = folding distortion
- Sweeping motion with hand inferiorly down back of thigh = posterior thigh tightness triggerband
- Gripping motion with both hands over iliac crest = tectonic fixation of hip

Question #2. Answer: A
  Since the goal of treating chronic pain is to first make the injury acute, the initial treatment in a chronic low back pain case such as this is to break the fascial adhesions and correct the triggerbands. A secondary reason is that the pulling pain down the posterior thigh is his primary complaint.

Question #3. Answer: E
  The chair technique is the most effective and easiest folding technique for low back pain to be done in the office setting. Note that inversion therapy is generally reserved for complex folding injuries or those that fail chair technique; traction is likely to be ineffective since it only unfolds in one plane; and wall technique is best utilized for lower thoracic unfolding injuries.

Question #4. Answer: E
  Frogleg and reverse frogleg manipulations are the most effective of all the tectonic techniques for the hip. Note that slow tectonic pump and the whip technique are generally reserved for hip tectonic fixations that don't initially respond to frogleg and reverse frogleg manipulations; the plunger is currently not powerful enough to circulate fluid deep in the hip joint; and the Kirksville crunch (a.k.a. dog technique) is utilized for thoracic (and on rare occasions lumbar) facet, not hip, tectonic fixations.

Question #5. Answer: C
  In the fascial distortion model the definition of chronic is entirely anatomical, (i.e., there are fascial adhesions) rather than temporal (i.e., length of time of symptoms).

Question #6. Answer: D
  It was ten years ago that Mr. W. began complaining of symptoms of a triggerband, so it was likely to be shortly thereafter that the adhesions formed.

Question #7. Answer: A
  Although we don't know the actual mechanism of injury, we can be confident that the initial pathology was a folding distortion of the lumbar spine. This can be assumed since tectonic fixations of the hip generally occur secondary to another principal fascial distortion type; and that the triggerband symptoms didn't occur until the last ten years.

Note that choice B and C cause folding distortions of the hip (unfolding and refolding, respectively). Although *overuse syndrome** (choice D) is a common medical diagnosis, it doesn't describe the underlying pathology, and fallaciously implies that reducing or eliminating the offending behavior will somehow correct the anatomical injury.

*An accomplished amateur female long-distance runner came to the office complaining of pain in her right lower leg whenever she ran more than five miles. Hearing about overuse syndrome she stated, "I think I am running too far on that leg." The reply given back was "How far are you running on the other leg?"

Case History #4 Osteoarthritic Knee Pain in a 71 Year Old Woman

History: No known injury to this woman with debilitating pain in both of her knees secondary to severe osteoarthritis. Her orthopedist sent her for orthopathic treatments when she refused bilateral knee replacement surgery.

Symptoms: Aching deep in both knees
Knees feel weak and give out, falls frequently
Has to use cane

Body Language: Squeezes knees with hands

Physical Exam: Walks slowly and awkwardly. Rises from chair with difficulty. Squatting ability is minimal. The knee joints themselves are enlarged and deformed. There is no point tenderness, no obvious swelling, redness, or warmth.

X-rays: Not reviewed

Orthopedic Diagnosis: Severe osteoarthritis of knees

Discussion Topic: Body language

Case History #4

Discussion: Although Ms. E.'s condition is orthopedically considered to be osteoarthritis, it can still be orthopathically assessed in the same manner as any other injury. In her case, the combination of an aching pain deep in the joint along with the body language of squeezing the knees is strongly suggestive of the presence of folding distortions.

Before Ms. E. was treated with folding technique, each of the knee joints were first compressed and then tractioned. It was determined that the pain could be magnified by pushing on the heel of the foot and driving the tibia into the distal femur. Likewise it was determined that pulling the foot and leg away from the knee decreased the discomfort. Because of these two findings, she was treated with an aggressive unfolding technique on each knee, which resulted in a significant decrease in symptoms, a normal gait, an improved ability to squat, and no need for the cane.

Ms. E. continues to be treated monthly.

Case History #5 Heel Pain in an 11 Year Old Boy

Chief Complaint: Bilateral heel pain x 2 years

History: J. is a young man who complained of pain in both of his heels for the past two years. Despite taking anti-inflammatory medicines and refraining from running, he continued to immediately limp whenever he participated in any fast-paced ambulatory activities.

Body Language: Sweeping motion with index and middle finger from calcaneus along plantar fascia to base of toes

PE: Normal arch of foot, no limp with walking, no point tenderness

X-ray Interpretation: Normal (done previously)

Orthopedic Diagnosis: Plantar fasciitis

Orthopathic Diagnosis: Triggerband plantar fasciitis

Discussion Topic: Plantar fasciitis

Case History #5

Discussion: J. was treated with triggerband technique from the triggerband starting point (at the junction of the calcaneus and plantar fascia) to the metatarsal/phalangeal joint. Since his injury was both acute (no adhesions) and superficial, the treatment itself was relatively painless. However, be aware that triggerbands of the plantar fascia can occur at varying depths with deeper layer distortions requiring more skill and thumb strength on the part of the physician.

Following the first triggerband treatment each of the feet were manipulated. This corrected the tectonic fixations which occurred secondary to diminished fascial fluid circulation due to the restrictive effect of long-standing triggerbands.

Immediately following the first treatment J. was able to run without pain. Re-treatment was done in two days, and an inquiry two months later found him to be symptom-free and fully participating in sports including all running activities.

Note that continuum distortions also can be the cause of plantar fasciitis. These present as pinpoint pain on the plantar aspect of the calcaneus. Body language consists of pointing to a spot of pain with one finger. Treatment is with continuum technique (i.e., application of direct pressure by the thumb into the most tender spot of discomfort and holding it until the transition zone shifts). This treatment generally involves a great deal of strength and stamina on the part of the physician and the all-or-none principle should not be forgotten — letting up before the release will result in a wasted effort by the orthopath.

With plantar fasciitis involving both triggerbands and continuum distortions, triggerbands should be treated first.

Case History #6 Upper Arm Pain Following Flu Shot

Chief Complaint: Left upper arm pain x 2 days

History: Ms. S., a 46 year old woman who was being treated for bilateral carpal tunnel syndrome, mentioned that she had pain in her left upper arm from a flu shot she received the day before. When asked to show exactly where it hurt, she responded by squeezing her upper arm with her right index finger and thumb around the injection site.

Orthopedic Diagnosis: Muscle contusion (bruise)

Discussion Topic: Orthopathic interpretation

Case History #7 Low Back Pain in a Woman with Multiple Compression Fractures

Chief Complaint: Low back pain x 20 years

History: Ms. H. was injured in a horseback riding accident 20 years ago, and sustained compression fractures of all five lumbar vertebrae. She spent three weeks in the hospital and gradually her symptoms began to diminish. In 1996 there were two exacerbations of her back pain after lifting household items. Because of her continuing pain, Ms. H. said that her neurosurgeon recommended an operation.

Symptoms: Pain deep in the spine
    Pulling pain from L1 to L5

Body Language: Sweeping motion with fingers from L1 to L5
    Shoves fist into lumbar vertebrae

Orthopathic Impression: Chronic low back pain secondary to compression fractures

Discussion Topic: Orthopathic treatment

Case History #6
Discussion: In the fascial distortion model the body language of squeezing or pinching the tissues is strongly suggestive of a cylinder distortion. Ms. S. was treated with double thumb cylinder technique which eliminated her discomfort.

Often with injections (particularly tetanus shots) the cylinder fascia becomes tangled; first by the needle which either severs or shoves the cylinder coils on top of one another, and then by the introduction of injected fluid whose volume physically displaces the coils from below.

In some instances a tetanus shot may result in a person losing motion in the entire arm or shoulder. On the Orthopathic Flow Chart of the Acutely Sore Shoulder it can be seen that when there is global loss of motion (i.e., abduction, and external and internal rotation are affected) accompanied by pain in the upper arm, this signifies that the underlying injury is a cylinder distortion. And since cylinder technique is designed to correct the anatomical cause of the injury, restoration of motion is expected with the treatment.

Case History #7
Discussion: Ms. H.'s symptoms are considered to originate from two sources: triggerbands with adhesions (making it chronic), and folding distortions of the lumbar spine. Therefore the initial office visit consisted of triggerband technique and a gentle folding manipulation in the chair. Since compression fractures can be thought of as a refolding injury to the osseous matrix, a slight compression force was applied during chair technique.

Then a hallelujah maneuver (standing lift technique) was done. This was initiated to correct the associated unfolding distortions that occurred both when she fell off the horse (but before she hit the ground) and from the two bending-forward injuries she had at home.

Over the next two months Ms. H. was treated seven more times in the office but also received inversion therapy (both inversion traction and ball therapy) to correct the array of multidirectional unfolding and refolding distortions. At the time of discharge and in follow-up inquiries, she remained pain free.

Case History #8 Fibromyalgia in a 45 Year Old Woman

Chief Complaint: Right upper back pain x 3 years (no known injury)

History: Ms. S. complains of pain in the right upper back just lateral to the spine and one inch medial to the medial border of the scapula. In addition, she complains of deep aching in the thoracic spine that is aggravated by standing.

Social History: Works at the post office

X-rays: Reportedly normal

Past Treatments: Medicines and physical therapy — "Didn't make a lot of difference"

Physical Exam: No point tenderness, normal shoulder movement, normal thoracic motion, normal reflexes

Orthopedic Diagnosis: "My doctor told me I have fibromyalgia"

Discussion Topic: Sequence of orthopathic interventions

Case History #8
Discussion: Orthopathically a typical treatment sequence in a so-called fibromyalgia patient would be:

1. Star triggerband
2. Star folding
3. Upper trapezius triggerband (if present)
4. Posterior shoulder triggerband pathway (if present)
5. SCHTP (if present)
6. Wall technique
7. First rib (refolding)
8. Kirksville crunch
9. Hallelujah maneuver

However, in this case there seemed to be only two primary distortions involved:
1. Star folding distortion
2. Lower thoracic folding distortions

Therefore Ms. S. would probably have done well with treatment of the star folding (unfolding of the intercostal membrane at the star triggerband starting point), followed by wall technique for the long-standing lower thoracic unfolding distortions. However, since over time other distortions may form secondary to the two major distortions, it is reasonable to take an additional ten or fifteen minutes and complete the entire sequence of treatments.

Note that in the fascial distortion model the term *fibromyalgia* does not imply that the injury is permanent or incurable.

Case History #9 Sprained Ankle in a 26 Year Old Woman

Chief Complaint: Left ankle pain x 7 days

History: Ms. S. is a nurse whose ankle buckled outward as she stepped part way off the edge of a porch. There was immediate pain and swelling. At the Emergency Department of the hospital where she works, an x-ray was taken (interpreted as negative), a "huge bandage" was applied, and she was put on crutches. The following day Ms. S was told by her physician to "stay off" the ankle and if not better to see an orthopedist.

Body Language: Points to the lateral aspect of the ankle with one finger to show source of pain, but also indicates with a sweeping motion that there is a pulling discomfort from the heel down along the lateral foot.

Physical Exam:
    Lateral malleolar swelling and ecchymosis
    No point tenderness
    Unable to bear weight
    Dorsiflexion = 1/4 with stepping
    Diminished eversion and inversion

Orthopedic Diagnosis: Ankle sprain

Orthopathic Diagnosis:
1. Continuum ankle sprain
2. Triggerband foot sprain

Discussion Topic: Orthopathic treatment

Case History #9
Discussion:

This ankle/foot sprain combination is best treated in this order:
1. Anterior ankle continuum distortion
2. Lateral ankle continuum distortions
3. Lateral foot triggerbands

Ms. S. was treated on a Friday and was immediately able to bear weight, stand on her toes, and to walk without a limp. By the time she returned to work later that afternoon almost all of the swelling was gone (re-establishment of the fascial fluid transport network). She was re-checked in the office on Monday and a gentle unfolding manipulation of the ankle was done. At the time of discharge she was completely asymptomatic.

Case History #10 Upper Arm Pain in a 67 Year Old Man

History: Mr. W. is a gentleman who complained of diffuse pain in the upper arm after injuring his right shoulder one week ago. On abduction he could raise the arm to only 120°, external rotation was grossly normal but painful, and internal rotation demonstrated a 7-inch deficit compared to the opposite side.

Discussion Questions:
1. Mr. W. injured his shoulder by:
    A. Walking his large dog which yanked its chain when it chased a cat
    B. Doing the backstroke swimming
    C. Slipping on the ice and jamming the head of his humerus into the glenoid fossa
    D. Performing chin-ups on a bar that he recently installed across his bedroom door
    E. Playing fetch with his neighbor's dog

2. Mr. W. did great with the first treatment and after the second treatment two days later he was completely asymptomatic and had normal range of motion. Unfortunately, three days later he returned to the office with the same symptoms, although his range of motion remained normal. What happened?
    A. He put heat on it
    B. He put ice on it
    C. His wife ace-wrapped an ice bag to his upper arm, and then he fell asleep on the sofa watching TV
    D. He had only pretended to feel better before
    E. The previous treatment failed because the diagnosis was wrong
    F. The treatment given was not expected to last and he missed his next office visit

3. Therefore Mr. W. was:
    A. Reassured but not treated (his behavior suggested that there was a strong emotional component to his complaints which should not be encouraged)
    B. Considered to have failed treatment so an MRI was ordered to rule out a rotator cuff tear
    C. Treated with triggerband technique and OMT of the shoulder
    D. Given an injection of cortisone and an analgesic medicine
    E. Arm ace-wrapped and placed in a sling
    F. Re-treated in a similar fashion as the previous treatment

Case History #10
Discussion:

Question #1. Answer: B
When performing the backstroke, Mr. W. extended and torqued his upper arm which tangled the superficial cylinder fascia. Answers A and E would likely result in unfolding distortions whereas Answer C would cause a refolding. Performing chin-ups (Answer D) involves no torque so wouldn't cause cylinders but could cause unfoldings or refoldings.

Question #2. Answer: C
Note that the reason Mr. W. felt so well after the first two treatments was that anatomically the injury was corrected. The only way he could have similar symptoms would be to have another injury that caused more cylinders. In this case more cylinders were formed when the ice melted and gravity pulled and torqued the bag downward which twisted and torqued the ace wrap and the underlying cylinder fascia.

Question #3. Answer: F
His new injury is a cylinder distortion so the treatment should again be cylinder technique.

Case History #11 Shoulder Pain in a 42 Year Old Woman

Chief Complaint: Pain deep in right shoulder x 3 months

History: Ms. M. injured her right shoulder three months earlier from slipping on a deodorant container that had inadvertently fallen in the aisle of a large department store. On impact the right shoulder and elbow were tucked against her side and took the brunt of the force from the fall. Immediately thereafter, Ms. M. felt somewhat disheveled but continued on with her day until it became apparent at lunch that there was a problem — she couldn't lift a coffee cup to her mouth.

The following day Ms. M. was sent by her doctor's physician assistant for evaluation by an orthopedic surgeon. Unfortunately, the MRI he ordered could not be performed because of the patient's claustrophobia. So instead, an injection was made into the shoulder which relieved a significant amount of the discomfort, suggesting to the orthopedist (according to Ms. M.) that there was an impingement syndrome. After three months of conservative care with no subjective or objective improvement, Ms. M. was scheduled for surgical excision of the lateral portion of her right clavicle.

Physical Exam:

	Before Orthopathic Treatment	After 1st Orthopathic Treatment
Abduction:	90° (50 % speed)	180° (normal speed)
External rotation:	awkward	normal
Internal rotation:	9" above waist line	12" above waist line (14" after 2nd treatment)

Discussion Topic: Orthopathic treatment sequence and goals

Case History #11

Discussion: The mechanism of accident and description of discomfort deep in the shoulder joint are strongly suggestive that the underlying fascial injury is a folding distortion. However, folding distortions on their own (with the exception of dislocations) don't cause significant loss of abduction. Therefore, there had to be another distortion (at least) involved to account for the loss of abduction (which in her case was the supraclavicular herniated triggerpoint). Note that the following approach resulted in a rapid recovery.

Treatment sequence and goals:

1. Restore abduction (treat SCHTP, and anterior and posterior shoulder triggerband pathways, if involved)
2. Restore speed of external rotation (treat anterior and posterior pathways and continuum distortions, if present)
3. Restore internal rotation and eliminate pain deep in shoulder (treat with refolding technique: accomplished by placing the shoulder and elbow in the same position as injury coupled with compression/thrust manipulation)

Case History #12 Chest Wall Pain in a 25 Year Old Man

History: Mr. G. injured his chest one year before while lifting a cast iron bathtub. Two days after the injury he had difficulty breathing and went to the Emergency Room where no pneumothorax or other medical emergent problem was identified. He gradually began to feel better but seven months later aggravated the chest again when carrying generators during the ice storm. On the first office visit, he pointed with one finger to the pain on the left chest, but the right side discomfort could not be localized.

Orthopedic Diagnosis: Chest wall pain (costochondritis)

Discussion Topic: Chest wall pain

Case History #13 Shoulder Pain in a 43 Year Old Woman

History: This woman complained of aching deep in the left shoulder "socket" for the past two days after being bucked off her horse and dragged on the ground by the reins. Pain was present with motion of the shoulder, but absent when the arm rested at her side.

Physical Exam:
    Normal gross abduction, stepping present
    Normal external rotation
    Internal rotation – total height equal on left and right, speed 1/4 on left, hand direction 60° bilaterally
    No point tenderness

Impression: Folding shoulder strain

Discussion Topic: Subtle signs of restricted shoulder motion

Case History #12

Discussion: Chest wall pain is generally due to both triggerbands and continuum distortions. In some instances folding distortions of the ribs and cylinder distortions may also be involved. In the case of Mr. G., he was treated first with triggerband technique followed by continuum technique and then folding/thrusting manipulation. The vagueness of his symptoms on the right side of the chest is almost certainly due to the adhesions disrupting mechanical sensory input. His chest pain was almost completely resolved after the first three sessions. However, four additional treatments were needed before the diagnosis of *chronic chest wall pain – resolved* could be made.

Case History #13

Discussion: Although abduction, external rotation, and internal rotation were grossly equivalent to the opposite shoulder, the subtle signs of stepping, hand direction, and speed indicated that there were significant underlying anatomical restrictions.

Treatment #1:
    Folding technique (unfolding) of left shoulder
        Result: 6" gain in total height
        Normal speed
        No stepping
        Vertical hand direction

Treatment #2:
    Recheck (two days later): Restored motion retained
        Slight pain in spot over anterior shoulder with extreme external rotation, treated with continuum technique

Note that following treatment the left shoulder had superior motion to the right; meaning that sometime in the past the right shoulder also had been injured.

Case History #14 Post-Stroke Spastic Paralysis Patient

History: Mr. C. is a 58 year old gentleman who suffered a stroke two years before coming to the office. He had diminished vision, right lower extremity spasticity, and spastic paralysis of the right upper extremity.

Discussion Questions:
1. Mr. C.'s main complaint is:
   A. Paralysis
   B. Spasm
   C. Pain
2. In looking at his spastic paralysis orthopathically, we envision his condition as:
   A. A central nervous system insult with uncontrollable neurological output
   B. Chronic, incurable, and permanent
   C. Consisting of multitudes of fascial distortions which peripherally disrupt electrical flow and physically restrict movement
3. Expected distortions of the frozen right shoulder include:
   A. SCHTP
   B. Triggerbands
   C. Adhesions
   D. Continuum distortions
   E. Folding distortions
   F. Cylinder distortions
   G. Tectonic Fixations
   H. All of the above
4. During his first office visit, shoulder abduction increased from 90° to 180°. The treatments most responsible for this improvement were:
   A. OMT to the neck and shoulder
   B. Anterior and posterior triggerband pathways and the SCHTP
   C. Continuum technique of the shoulder
   D. Cylinder technique of the upper arm
5. The loss of proprioception of the upper extremity (he couldn't tell where his hand was unless he looked at it) was solved within several treatments by utilizing:
   A. Muscle energy technique
   B. OMT to the neck
   C. Triggerband and cylinder technique
   D. Aggressive proprioceptive training with a skilled physical therapist
6. The numbness, decreased sensation, and loss of balance in the lower extremity was predominantly secondary to:
   A. A tectonic fixation of the hip
   B. Bull's-eye herniated triggerpoint
   C. Continuum distortions of the sacroiliac joint
   D. Folding distortions of the intermuscular septum
   E. Triggerbands of the iliotibial tract
   F. Cylinder distortions of the thigh

Case History #14
Discussion:

Question #1. Answer C
For most PSSPP's with long-standing symptoms, the number one reason for seeking treatment is pain. This is true not only because pain is the most irritating aspect of their disability but because they don't even consider the prospect that spasticity or paralysis can be helped.

Question #2. Answer C
The intent of treatment is therefore to:
* Remove anatomical restrictions which physically impede muscle contractions and joint movements
* Allow for proper distribution of neurological flow to target muscles

Question #3. Answer H
The four mechanisms by which multitudes of fascial distortions occur in PSSPP's are:
* Decreased muscle tone in the initial flaccid state allows fascial tissues to crumple, wrinkle, and overfold
* Diminished synovial fluid circulation in the flaccid state coupled with physical restriction of joint movement leads to tectonic fixations
* Return of neurologic flow to the flaccid limb causes chaotic muscle contractions which tear apart fascial fibers, tangle cylindric coils, push underlying tissue through adjacent fascial planes, shift osseous components into ligamental and tendon transition zones, and unfold and refold interosseous membranes into pathological orientations
* Fascial distortion generation from pre-existing fascial distortions (see Chapter 9)

Question #4. Answer B
The SCHTP and the anterior and posterior triggerband pathways are always the most likely distortions responsible for impaired abduction. Note that cylinder distortions cause global loss of motion in acute sore shoulders, and that continuum distortions generally don't affect abduction. Answer A (OMT to the neck and shoulder) is a generic description that doesn't state what anatomical distortion is present or physically how that distortion is engaged by the treatment.

Question #5. Answer C
Triggerbands and cylinder distortions are generally the fascial culprits in altered proprioception; therefore triggerband and cylinder techniques are treatments of choice.

Question #6. Answer E
Triggerbands of the iliotibial tract (the largest fascial band in the body) are notorious for causing numbness, decreased sensation, and loss of balance in the lower extremity.

Case History #15 Upper Back Pain in a 21 Year Old Woman

Outline of Events: Motor vehicle accident four months ago
No obvious initial injuries
Upper back pain started one hour later
Seen by family doctor 2 days later
Treated by two chiropractors (13 visits)
Twenty physical therapy sessions
Four months later still complains of upper back pain

Orthopedic Diagnosis: Thoracic strain

Orthopathic Approach:
1. Review events of accident and consider anatomical ramifications
2. Observe body language
3. Decipher verbal complaints
4. Physical examination
5. Orthopathic diagnosis
6. Treat (correct involved fascial distortions)

Motor Vehicle Accident:
Patient driver of car stopped at signal
Rear-ended by another vehicle of unknown speed
At instant of impact she was reaching downward with right hand to change radio station, right shoulder was forward with forearm supinated
Seatbelt and shoulder harness fastened
Shoulder harness lax prior to collision
No air bag

Body Language:
1. Grasps right supraclavicular area with left hand and pushes fingers into fossa
2. Tugs superiorly on upper thoracic spinous processes with fingers

Verbal Complaints:
1. Burning pain along right shoulder blade that pulls into neck
2. Denies shoulder complaints
3. "Tingling" in right upper extremity following prolonged sitting (last two weeks only)

Relevant Findings:
Normal neuro exam
Normal x-rays
Normal neck and thoracic exam
5" deficit on internal rotation of right shoulder compared to left

Orthopathic Diagnosis: Shoulder strain secondary to: 1. SCHTP, 2. Star triggerband, 3. Folding distortions of upper back, 4. Cylinder distortion of right upper extremity.

Discussion Topic: Given the specific events of the motor vehicle accident and other relevant factors, relate the physical forces of injury to the formation of the anatomical distortions.

Case History #15
Discussion: The initial distortions formed at impact as the thorax was rammed forward (because she was flexed at the waist the force is directed anatomically superiorly) while the harness restrained the shoulder. This combination of pushing the thorax forward (i.e., superiorly) coupled with immobilization of the shoulder, widened the supraclavicular fossa and physically forced underlying tissue through the fascial plane (formation of SCHTP).

The twisted thorax and restrained shoulder also introduced uneven forces into the horizontal plane and sheared apart fascial fibers along the star triggerband pathway.

During the collision, the car and driver were thrust forward, unfolding the thoracic paravertebral fascia superiorly (since she was bent forward), which then refolded contorted (since she was also twisted).

The delayed complaint of tingling throughout the entire upper extremity is, within the FDM, the result of cylinder distortions. In her case the cylinder coils of the upper extremity tangled from the uneven tugging effect caused by the functional shortening of fibers associated with pre-existing fascial distortions.

Case History #16 Ankle Pain in a 39 Year Old Woman

Chief Complaint: Left ankle pain x 33 years

History: Ankle fracture at age 6
No surgery
Frequent ankle sprains (approximately one per year)
Walks upstairs with limp
Bi-malleolar swelling following exertion
Aching deep in joint

Physical Exam: Mild pes planus bilaterally
Mild bi-malleolar and foot swelling
No point tenderness
Unable to stand on toes of left foot
Normal dorsiflexion
No obvious limp

Orthopedic Diagnosis: Chronic ankle pain

Orthopathic Diagnosis: Long-standing acute folding ankle sprain

Treatment:
#1 Unfolding technique done — "I feel a lot better"
#2 (5 days later) No swelling
Patient says she's been "Beating on it," but no pain
Unfolding technique repeated
#3 (2 weeks later) "99% better"
Unfolding technique repeated

Phone Inquiry (15 months later) No swelling, no aching — "I can still walk on my toes, go up steps without pain. . . I don't think about it anymore"

Discussion Topic: Body language

Case History #16
Discussion: The body language of folding distortions of the ankle consists of:

Unfolding: Gently grasps the ankle, distal leg, or foot
Refolding: Same as above, plus a sideways pushing sweep with the fingers back and forth across the top of the ankle

The orthopathic pathology of this particular injury was solely an unfolding distortion. The body language actually observed was grasping the ankle with the hand and giving it a slight squeeze with the fingers. Note that the fact that the injury was long-standing does not change the body language or slow the rate of response to the treatments. If the injury had been chronic, i.e., triggerbands with adhesions had formed, then for a successful outcome it would have been necessary to employ triggerband technique before utilizing folding technique.

Case History #17 Left Lower Extremity Weakness in a Woman with Post-Polio Syndrome

History: 51 year old woman with history of profound left lower extremity weakness since early teenage years. Patient had polio at age 3 with apparent recovery. However, ten years later she experienced significant weakness in her left lower extremity. The initial diagnosis made was multiple sclerosis, but over the next several years was changed to post-polio syndrome. Last neurological exam was four years ago.

Past Medical History:
- Polio
- Post-polio syndrome
- Fibromyalgia
- Bilateral frozen shoulders
- Chronic low back pain
- Short left leg
- Bilateral carpal tunnel syndrome

Past Surgical History: Foot surgery x 2 on the left (single and then triple fusions)

Physical Exam: Prominent atrophy and weakness noted in left lower extremity. A 1 1/4" lift is present on the left shoe. The hip is unable to actively flex more than 20° in the standing position. Gait is abnormal with left foot barely able to clear the floor when stepping. Positioned in supine with the knee passively flexed, the patient is unable to actively hold the knee in midline (floppy leg).

Impression: Post-polio syndrome with left lower extremity weakness secondary to a tectonic fixation of the hip

Plan: Tectonic technique of the hip (one treatment was done in the supine position). The hip was placed into an extreme Patrick-Fabere position and a thrust was made into the restriction. An impressive slide-clunk was both heard and felt. Then the hip was placed into a reverse Patrick-Fabere position and a thrust in the opposite direction was made. This resulted in a smaller audible clunk.

Results:
    Hip flexion in the standing position improved to above 90°
    Strength and speed of motion looked normal
    Gait was more fluid and less awkward
    In the supine position with the knee flexed, there was coordinated abduction and adduction of the hip without the floppy leg phenomena
    For the first time in her life she was able to get into her car without having to lift her thigh with her hands. She did this six consecutive times with little obvious strain and no apparent fatigue.

Discussion Topic: Mechanism of formation of tectonic fixation

Case History #17

Discussion: In the fascial distortion model, post-polio syndrome as well as cerebral palsy, strokes, multiple sclerosis, and muscular dystrophy are envisioned as neurological disabilities compounded by fascial distortions (collectively designated as neuro/fascial conditions). In this woman's case it was not the weakness of the muscles that kept her from lifting her thigh, it was the tectonic fixation of the head of the femur on the acetabulum which locked the thigh to the hip. Once the fixation was broken the huge amounts of energy which were previously needed to force the head of the femur along the acetabulum to raise the thigh were no longer necessary. The apparent increase in muscular strength following the treatment results from the relatively limited neurological input from the brain now being focused on muscular motion rather than having it wasted on femoral drag.

In this particular case it is thought that the tectonic fixation itself resulted from the post-polio syndrome which initially caused diminished neurological input to the joint. The decreased neurological input resulted in decreased muscular motion of the thigh which eventually diminished synovial fluid circulation. Over time pockets of devitalized fluid formed between the two abutting surfaces of the joint and, in a sudden event during her teenage years, the polarity shifted so that the surfaces instantaneously became attracted to each other (i.e., changed from the normal repulsive state to the attracted state).

Tectonic technique broke the fixation and forced the joint surfaces to slide on each other. This allowed the synovial fluid to re-circulate which reversed the polarity. The surfaces of the joint then once again repelled each other which reduced the dragging of the femoral head on the acetabulum.

Although in post-polio syndrome the neurological supply to the affected limb is expected to be far less than normal, it is typically more than sufficient for simple tasks such as lifting the thigh and walking with a normal gait. However, with the presence of concurrent fascial distortions the neuro supply becomes functionally inadequate. Elimination of the distortion then results in a clinically significant improvement in both motion and strength.

Note: Follow-up on this patient seven months later revealed that motion and strength continued to improve. This was evident by her ability to:
1. Stand alone on the left leg for 20 seconds
2. Lift her left foot up and place it on the treatment chair

Case History #18 Frozen Shoulder/Reflex Sympathetic Dystrophy-Like Symptoms in a 38 Year Old Woman

Ms. T. has two significant complaints:
1. Frozen left shoulder
2. Excruciating tenderness of the left shoulder and upper back

Relevant Facts:
- Onset 1 1/2 years ago
- Progressive increase in pain
- No known injury
- Severe asthma x 15 years (unable to receive anesthesia)
- Shoulder injection x 1 (no subjective change)
- Physical therapy not done (therapists refused to treat due to patients inability to tolerate light physical contact including ultrasound or electrical stimulation)
- MRI of shoulder and upper thoracic area reported as normal

Physical Exam:
- Audible wheezing
- Abduction = 100° with anterior rotation
- External rotation = slow, stepping
- Internal rotation = 1/4 speed, 4" above waist line (5" deficit compared to right shoulder)
- Thoracic/shoulder soft tissue: right = not tender, left = excruciatingly tender

Orthopathic Impression:
1. Frozen shoulder secondary to tectonic fixation
2. Reflex sympathetic dystrophy-like symptoms secondary to cylinder distortions

Discussion Questions:
1. Ms. T. was extremely tender to the touch, so much so that even tapping her upper back with a pencil brought tears to her eyes. This exquisite pain was due to:
   A. An alteration of the fascial mechanical sensory system (the fascial fibers are *out of tune*)
   B. A shift in the physiological continuum
   C. A neuroma of the spinal cord
   D. A somatic dysfunction of the autonomic nervous system causing a visceral-somatic response
2. Ms. T. did well with her treatments and was discharged two weeks later (total of five visits) with a final diagnosis of 1. Frozen shoulder – resolved, and 2. Reflex sympathetic dystrophy – resolved. The cylinder distortions which contributed to the reflex sympathetic dystrophy symptoms were formed by:
   A. Her original injury (which is unknown)
   B. The MRI disrupting the energy field of the fascia
   C. The anti-inflammatory medicines she had been taking blocking fascial fluid transport (road-block effect)
   D. Shortened fascial bands (triggerbands) pulling unevenly on cylindrical superficial fascia causing them to tangle

Case History #18
Discussion:

Question #1 Answer A
Within the FDM, the bizarre and oftentimes extreme sensory findings of reflex sympathetic dystrophy are the result of cylinder distortions. The problem in interpreting the garbled sensory input from the distorted fascial network is comparable in difficulty to the challenge of recognizing the melody from the *Blue Danube* when the violin section of the orchestra is playing with instruments hopelessly out of tune.

Question #2 Answer D
Ms. T.'s extreme palpatory tenderness developed after the shoulder had become frozen. The cylinder distortions were therefore not part of the initial injury but developed secondary to the uneven pull of pre-existing triggerbands on the superficial fascial coils.

The development of this injury occurred in several steps, so to the patient there is no one obvious initial incident:
- Step 1: Triggerbands and SCHTP formed from forces of initial injury (unknown)
- Step 2: Tectonic fixations developed when the capsule and humeral head surfaces magnetically attracted each other (secondary to the SCHTP and triggerbands limiting shoulder motion which diminished synovial fluid circulation and changed the electrical polarity)
- Step 3: The tectonic fixation unevenly limited motion so that when the shoulder forcibly moved, the shortened fascial fibers torqued specific portions of cylindrical coils

Treatment Steps:
1. Correct the SCHTP and triggerbands
2. Slow tectonic pump followed by frogleg and reverse frogleg tectonic technique
3. Squeegee cylinder technique for broad areas that elicit bizarre or painful tactile responses, and double thumb cylinder technique for smaller or more defined patches of discomfort

Case History #19 Frozen Shoulder in a 45 Year Old Woman

History: Ms. D. developed a painful right shoulder 10 months ago after spending four days in bed with asthma during an ice storm. Her family doctor noted that her shoulder movement was normal and prescribed a home exercise program. At recheck in two weeks, Ms. D. had significant loss of shoulder motion and marked increase in pain. An x-ray was taken which was interpreted as normal.

Medications and physical therapy (heat, ultrasound, pendulum swinging, shoulder shrugs, and pulleys) were begun, and at recheck one month later flexion had improved to 60°. Following a normal MRI the patient was referred for orthopathic manipulation.

Past Medical History:
  Severe extrinsic asthma
  No previous shoulder injury
  Multiple allergies to broad groups of medicines including anesthetics
  Medically unable to tolerate surgery

Social History: Formerly a teacher
          Disabled from asthma

Physical Exam:
  Severe wheezing with increased respiratory rate
  Abduction: 70° (with anterior rotation of shoulder)
  Flexion: 80°
  External rotation: cannot attain position
  Internal rotation: below sacroiliac joint
  Painful active and passive motion

Orthopathic Impression: Frozen shoulder secondary to tectonic fixation

Outcome After 35 Orthopathic Treatments:
  Abduction: 170°
  External rotation: normal
  Internal rotation: 6" above waistline
  Flexion: 170°
  Near ability to circumduct shoulder
  Painless active and passive range of motion

Discussion Topic: Number of treatments

Case History #19

Discussion: The large number of treatment sessions is generally not acceptable for the following reasons:
1. It demonstrates lack of results and clear-cut objectives
2. What is accomplished on the thirtieth office visit can most often be done on the sixth, third, or even first visit
3. It requires an excessive amount of travel and time on the part of the patient
4. It diminishes confidence in the physician
5. It means that an anatomical change is not being made

The large number of sessions for Ms. D. was in part due to:
1. Respiratory condition was exacerbated by the physical nature of the therapy which limited the length and aggressiveness of each session
2. The sluggishness of the synovial fluid of the joint
3. Technical failure of the employed tectonic technique

The sluggishness of the synovial fluid was almost certainly due to its viscosity. If it had been sampled, we likely would have seen a cottage cheese-like material instead of clear, colorless, and water-like fluid. Sampling, however, was not an option in this case for three reasons: 1. Ms. D. is allergic to multiple anesthetics and antibiotics (which limits our ability to shield her from the pain of the procedure and the medical response to complications); 2. The thick fluid aspirates poorly; and 3. From a respiratory perspective, the procedure itself could trigger a bout of status asthmaticus.

However, the primary reason for the treatment failing was that the tectonic techniques used at that time were either designed to slide the capsule or force synovial fluid quickly between the fixated surfaces. Half-way through the course of treatment, slow tectonic pump was developed to not only force fluid through the joint but to give the thickened fluid sufficient time to circulate between the fixated surfaces before being pumped again. And clinically, once "the pump" was introduced into the treatment process Ms. D. immediately showed marked increase in both active and passive motion.

Note that a near-future orthopathic approach currently under consideration for correcting pronounced shoulder tectonic fixations involves:
1. Inserting a needle into the joint and aspirating (and then discarding) as much of the thickened stagnant synovial fluid as possible
2. Trans-injecting (and then pumping back and forth) normal synovial fluid from the opposite shoulder or another unaffected joint into the tectonic joint

Case History #20 Spinal Stenosis in a 52 Year Old Man

Chief Complaints: Low back pain
Inability to walk long distances

History: Mr. B. complained of low back pain for the past year whenever he walked. The pain was predominantly in the right buttocks and thigh, but would spread to the left side if he continued to ambulate. His walking was limited to 500 feet, at which point he would have to sit and rest.

CT of Lumbar Spine – Impression:
1. Hypertrophic facet osteoarthritis with ligamentum flavum hypertrophy on the left at L5-S1 level, question left L5 radiculopathy
2. Mild broad-based disc bulges at L3-4 and L4-5 with mild central canal stenosis
3. There is no evidence for focal disc herniation on this examination

Medical Problems: Insulin dependent diabetes x 7 years
Vascular bypass surgery x 1 in the past
Coronary balloon angioplasty x 1 in the past

Neurosurgical Impression: Spinal stenosis

Neurosurgical Plan: Scheduled for surgery

Discussion Topic: Orthopathic approach to spinal stenosis

Case History #20
Discussion: In spinal stenosis, back pain is often the initial complaint followed by nerve compression symptoms of both lower extremities. Symptoms are exacerbated by exercise or lordosis and relieved by flexion of the spine. Persons at risk for spinal stenosis are those with decreased lateral recesses of the canal or decreased anterior-posterior dimensions of the spinal cord.

In the FDM the treatment approach for spinal stenosis is to anatomically unfold the paravertebral fascia which are constricting (either directly or indirectly) the spinal canal or surrounding structures. This is done primarily by two methods: 1. chair technique, and 2. inversion therapy. In either case, the primary corrective spinal position is traction and exaggerated flexion coupled with or without a superior directed lateral thrust.

Mr. B. was treated 10 times in the office and 11 times with inversion therapy (ball therapy and inversion traction). After the first office visit he felt substantially better, and after the third he ran 1/2 mile without any difficulty. At discharge he had no pain and no other symptoms of spinal stenosis. A phone inquiry for this book 15 months later found him to be asymptomatic and still walking and running without difficulty.

Case History #21 Elbow Pain in a 57 Year Old Man

Chief Complaint: Left elbow pain x 2 months

History: Mr. H. denies any known injury but thinks he could have strained his elbow pulling a boat onto a dock. His main complaint is tenderness of the lateral epicondyle where there is a specific point that if pushed on "makes me cry." In addition to point tenderness, he has tightness of the elbow joint, pulling pain along the proximal dorsal forearm, generalized discomfort below the elbow, and weakness in grip strength.

Physical Exam: No swelling
Normal range of motion
No redness
Tender spot of pain on lateral epicondyle
X-ray – not done

Orthopedic Impression: Lateral epicondylitis

Orthopathic Treatment #1: Tectonic technique (modified frogleg and reverse frogleg) was done to force the joint to slide and to subjectively reduce joint tightness. This was followed by continuum technique of "that spot of pain" on the lateral epicondyle. Together these two procedures eliminated the stiffness in the elbow and the point tenderness of the epicondyle.

Orthopathic Treatment #2: Although there were no complaints of elbow stiffness or spots of tenderness, three symptoms remained:
1. Pulling pain along the forearm
2. Below-the-elbow weakness
3. Diminished grip strength

Discussion Topic: Orthopathic etiology of diminished grip strength

Case History #21

Discussion: This gentleman had epicondylitis secondary to a continuum distortion of the lateral epicondyle, but also had a tectonic fixation of the elbow, and a triggerband of the interseptal membrane of the forearm. However, once these distortions were treated there was still an objective finding of diminished grip strength with an accompanying perception of forearm weakness. In the FDM, weakness of an extremity in the absence of pain signifies the presence of cylinder distortions. Treatment #2 therefore, was expanded to include Indian burn technique of the forearm and elbow which normalized grip strength and eliminated the sensation of forearm weakness.

However, Mr. H. then immediately experienced an entirely new sensation — tingling of the distal phalanx of the index finger. In the FDM the symptom of tingling (especially when associated with jumping) is a common clinical presentation of cylinder distortions (carpal tunnel syndrome is a better-known example). Mr. H.'s finger was treated with Indian burn technique by wrapping small gauze bandages around the distal and middle phalanx (to give a better grip) and tractioning apart the cylinder coils with a twisting force introduced from the orthopath's fingers. Note that in this procedure the treating hands are positioned so that the fingers of one hand grip the distal phalanx and twist it in one direction at the same time as the fingers of the other hand grasp the middle phalanx and twist it in the opposite direction. The torquing force is held until the tissue tautness lessens. The anticipated subjective response is elimination of the paraesthesia symptoms, which was the case with Mr. H.

Case History #22 Ankle Pain in an 80 Year Old Woman

History: An 80 year old woman injured her ankle 3 years ago. The incident occurred when she twisted it after arising from a long period of time sitting in a chair. She says that when she got up out of the chair her foot was "asleep" and she couldn't feel it hit the ground. She had immediate swelling, couldn't bear weight, and within a few days the lateral ankle was black and blue. X-ray revealed no fracture. Ms. H. complained that the ankle hurt intermittently deep in the lateral aspect of the joint.

Discussion Questions:
1. Her original injury is likely a _____.
   A. Triggerband
   B. Inverted continuum distortion
   C. Everted continuum distortion
   D. Unfolding distortion
   E. Refolding distortion
   F. Cylinder distortion
   G. Tectonic fixation

2. She was treated with the appropriate technique on the initial office visit and all of her original complaints completely abated. On recheck in two weeks she was doing well, and a second more aggressive treatment was done. Although she continued to be completely free of her original symptoms, she soon developed a totally new complaint . . . a vague discomfort in the distal leg. This seemingly new problem was due to:
   A. Increased fascial fluid transport
   B. Improved sensory perception
   C. The fact that the old problem was only partially corrected
   D. The treatment
   E. The emotional need of an elderly person for attention

3. The next step was therefore to:
   A. Reassure her
   B. Check for other signs of senility
   C. Re-treat in the same manner as the previous treatment
   D. Apply an ace wrap
   E. Use triggerband technique
   F. Use double thumb cylinder technique
   G. None of the above

4. In her case the symptoms are likely to reoccur:
   A. If she puts ice on the ankle
   B. If she wears the wrong shoes
   C. If she puts an ace wrap on it
   D. Over time
   E. All the above

Case History #22

5. The reason that her ankle hurt for so long was that:
   A. It had become chronic
   B. There was a stress fracture missed on the initial x-ray
   C. The shoes the podiatrist had her wear were aggravating the problem
   D. She put heat on it immediately following the injury
   E. She didn't rest it enough after it first became swollen
   F. She refused to walk on it for several weeks following the injury
   G. None of the above

Discussion:

Question #1. Answer E
   As her ankle hit the ground, the folding fascia was overcompressed.

Question #2. Answer D
   Although the refolding technique involved compression/thrust of the ankle, the fingers of the doctor inadvertently forced the cylinder coils in the leg to overlap each other. The formation of a cylinder distortion from a refolding treatment generally only occurs in individuals with delicate fascia (such as the elderly and those with connective tissue disorders).

Question #3. Answer F
   Double thumb cylinder technique is therapy of choice for cylinder distortions that are limited in size. Note: In an elderly person Indian burn should be avoided altogether, and squeegee technique is best employed to correct cylinder distortions that involve a large, broad area.

Question #4. Answer C
   If an ace wrap is torqued as it is applied, cylinder distortions can be created.

Question #5. Answer G
   The ankle continued to hurt because the anatomical injury (refolding distortion) had never been corrected.

Case History #23 Acute Abdominal Pain in a 62 Year Old Woman

Chief Complaint: Abdominal pain

History: This generally healthy woman, who was driving through town on vacation, presented to the Emergency Department with a complaint of several hours of progressing abdominal pain. The evening before she had entertained and there was no indication of illness. But at 0400 she was awakened with mid-back pain and shortly thereafter experienced nausea and epigastric discomfort. Later that morning she took 800 mg of ibuprofen and continued on her travels. However, she was soon forced by the pain to seek help at a local hospital.

Review of Symptoms: Denies fever, shortness of breath, chest pain, or diarrhea. Her last bowel movement was well formed and occurred the morning that her symptoms began. Ms. P. states she exercises regularly and "watches" her diet.

Past Medical History: Tonsillectomy and adenoidectomy as a child. She is a Gravida 4 Para 4 with four vaginal deliveries. Only surgery was dilation and curettage many years ago, with no other hospitalizations. Denies hypertension, diabetes, cancer, heart disease, or other illnesses.

Social History: She works as a nurse. Negative use of tobacco or illicit drugs. Alcohol intake is two mixed drinks per night with perhaps twice that consumed the past week. Ms. P. lives with her husband.

Physical Exam: Well-developed and well-nourished white female who appeared to be uncomfortable from her abdominal pain (rocks back and forth in bed). Alert and oriented times four. Skin is dry. No rash is visualized. Tongue is moist. No alcohol noticed on breath. Neck is not stiff. No scleral icterus. Heart is regular; lungs clear with unlabored respiration. Abdomen: soft, normal bowel sounds, no rebound or guarding, diffuse tenderness noted with localized points of pain deep in the abdominal cavity. Kidney punch is bilaterally negative.

Plan: Blood drawn and x-rays taken. Herniated triggerpoint therapy of the abdomen was performed with nearly complete elimination of pain. Following herniated triggerpoint therapy Ms. P. remained comfortable during her Emergency Room stay, so much so that she requested to be allowed to resume her vacation. However, laboratory and x-rays demonstrated the following:

    UA: Clear, negative glucose, +100 protein, 0-2 WBC's,
      specific gravity 1.025
    CBC: WBC = 11,400; H/H= 15.4 / 45.4; MCV = 96.4
    Glucose = 156, **Elytes** = normal, **GOT** = 392
    Total bili = 0.7, **GPT** =263, **Alk Phos** = 113, **LDH** = 409
    Cholesterol = 196, **Amylase** = 3048
    X-rays = No obvious obstruction or abnormal gas pattern

Discussion Topic: Medical diagnosis

Case History #23
Medical Diagnosis: Gallstone pancreatitis
                        Cholecystitis, cholelithiasis

Hospital Course: Ms. P. was admitted to the hospital with acute pancreatitis and was discharged eight days later. Ultrasound of the abdomen revealed an abnormal gallbladder with sludge and suspected gallstones. During her hospital stay she again developed abdominal pain and became febrile with a left shift. HIDA scan showed an open cystic duct with delayed emptying of the common duct. ERCP suggested clear common duct. Clinical impression by her physicians was that a gallstone had obstructed the duct and then passed. Several days before discharge a laparoscopic cholecystectomy was performed without complications. Patient was discharged in good condition, afebrile, eating well, and fully ambulatory.

Discussion: The high level of amylase (3048 with normal being 15-125) was strongly suggestive of pancreatitis. In the Emergency Room, herniated triggerpoint therapy was initiated as an adjunct medical treatment to relieve pain. However, it is possible that the treatment itself may have alleviated the obstruction by dislodging a stone (amylase the following day was 984 and three days later it dropped to 57).

Case History #24 Psoriatic Arthritis in a 43 Year Old Woman

Chief Complaint: Right hand pain and swelling

History: Ms. J. has a long history of psoriasis of the skin, but this last year has had an additional clinical manifestation of joint swelling and pain. The diagnosis of psoriatic arthritis was made by her rheumatologist who recommended treatment with methotrexate. However, because of the possible side effects of this chemotherapeutic agent, Ms. J. refused this option.

Minor Symptoms: Pain on bottom of foot
Left hand pain
Pain over medial aspect of right shoulder

Main Complaint: Swelling and pain of right hand, index and middle finger, with inability to make a fist, pick up coins, or use index and middle finger to button her blouse.

Physical Exam: Shoulders: bilateral normal abduction and external rotation. Internal rotation on left is normal speed, no flaring, with total height 12" above the waist. Internal rotation on right is 1/2 speed, three fingers of flaring, with total height 5" above the waist. Left hand makes normal grip, but there is erythema present at the tip of the distal phalanx of the third finger along with a noticeable deformity of the distal interphalangeal joint. The dorsum of right hand is markedly swollen particularly over the second and third metacarpal/phalangeal joints. The index and middle finger are unable to make a fist (index finger comes 1" from touching the thenar eminence; the middle finger is 2" shy). The middle finger has prominent swelling and tenderness in the proximal phalanx. The index finger is equally swollen. There is redness over distal posterior hand. Nails have pitting. Skin: patchy psoriatic lesions are noted on trunk.

Impression: 1. Psoriasis
2. Psoriatic arthritis
3. Partially frozen right shoulder
4. Right hand pain and swelling secondary to psoriatic arthritis

Discussion Topic: Treatment of psoriatic arthritic hand pain

Case History #24

Discussion: The pain and swelling of psoriatic arthritis is in many ways similar to the pain and swelling following a traumatic injury. On further questioning, Ms. J. gave a more detailed description of her right hand pain which included:
1. Diffuse vague discomfort on dorsum of hand
2. Deep aching in metacarpal/phalangeal and interphalangeal joints

Contemplating this presentation through the FDM, note:
1. Diffuse and non-specific pain is suggestive of cylinder distortions
2. Deep aching in joints, particularly associated with swelling extending to both sides of the joint, is suggestive of folding distortions

Therefore, the fascial pathology in this arthritic hand is considered to be cylinder and folding distortions.

Ms. J. was treated first with folding technique (unfolding manipulation) of the metacarpal/phalangeal joints (traction/thrust the finger away from the hand) followed by double thumb cylinder technique of the dorsum of the hand, and Indian burn cylinder technique of the forearm and fingers. At the time of discharge:
1. Right index finger could touch thenar eminence
2. Flexion of the middle finger was still 1/2" shy
3. Visible decrease in hand swelling

Also during that first office visit the right shoulder was treated with herniated triggerpoint therapy of the SCHTP. Her internal rotation total height improved 5 inches.

At recheck two days later Ms. J. could easily touch the thenar eminence with the index finger, but was still 1/2" away from doing so with the middle finger. Finger and hand swelling had decreased to "about half" what it had been prior to the initial office visit. The second treatment was similar to the first in that it consisted of folding and cylinder techniques. At discharge Ms. J. was able to make a non-painful fist with all her fingers. The change in finger and hand dexterity was most obvious to her as she buttoned her sweater and was able, for the first time in a year, to use her index and middle fingers in the process.

Note that the second visit did not involve the shoulder. Ms. J. felt that it was "back to normal" and another treatment "wasn't necessary." It is likely that the HTP of the shoulder was a separate injury unrelated to her psoriatic arthritis.

SECTION FOUR

ADDENDUM

SUMMARY OF COMMON ORTHOPATHIC CONDITIONS, BODY LANGUAGE, AND TREATMENTS

Condition	Body Language/ Description of Discomfort	Orthopathic Treatment
Headache/ Behind-the-Eye	Pushes thumb or finger tip into lacrimal bone	Triggerband technique from TMJ along the eyebrow to the lacrimal fossa, then gentle herniated triggerpoint therapy of tiny lacrimal HTP
Headache/ Occipital	Pushes and tugs on infra-occipital fascia with one or two fingers	Vigorous triggerband technique of peri-occipital fascia – treat from midline laterally
Headache/ Tension	1. Runs fingers along scalp	Triggerband technique along course of discomfort
	2. Pushes fingers into skull sutures	Refolding followed by unfolding technique (Note: Concurrent cranial technique facilitates fascial fluid circulation between fixated suture surfaces)
	3. Squeezes scalp	Double thumb cylinder technique of symptomatic scalp fascia
TMJ Pain	1. Rubs finger over TMJ	Triggerband technique along course of discomfort
	2. Points with finger to spot(s) of pain	Continuum technique
	3. Ache deep in joint, pain lessened with traction	Unfolding technique (doctor sits at end of table with patient supine, palms are placed over TMJ and the fingers are interlaced), traction/thrust force is directed along line of mandible
	4. Ache deep in joint, pain worse with traction	Refolding technique – direct compression/thrust of mandible superiorly and posteriorly into TMJ
	5. Stiffness	Neutral thrust tectonic manipulation of TMJ

Condition	Body Language/ Description of Discomfort	Orthopathic Treatment
Shoulder Pain	Pulling pain on front of shoulder	Triggerband technique of anterior shoulder pathway
	Pulling pain along back of shoulder	Triggerband technique of posterior shoulder pathway
	Pulling pain from upper back to neck	Triggerband technique of star
	Places palm of opposite hand over supraclavicular fossa	Herniated triggerpoint therapy of SCHTP
	Pain in spot(s)	Continuum technique
	Ache deep in joint, squeezes shoulder joint with opposite hand, tugs on hand	Unfolding technique (i.e., traction/thrust)
	Ache deep in joint, squeezes shoulder joint and pushes several fingers across humeral head	Refolding technique (i.e., compression/thrust)
	Squeezes upper arm with opposite hand	Double thumb cylinder technique
	Stiffness and pain with active movement, anterior rotation of shoulder with abduction	Slow tectonic pump followed by frogleg and reverse frogleg tectonic techniques
Upper Arm Pain	Sweeping motion with fingers along anterior upper arm	Triggerband technique of anterior shoulder pathway
	Sweeping motion with fingers along posterior upper arm	Triggerband technique of posterior shoulder pathway
	Squeezes localized portion of upper arm	Double thumb cylinder technique or squeegee technique of involved area

Condition	Body Language/ Description of Discomfort	Orthopathic Treatment
Upper Arm Pain	Repetitively squeezes multiple areas	Squeegee cylinder technique of entire upper arm
Elbow Pain	Sweeping motion of fingers over epicondyle	Triggerband technique
	Point tenderness on epicondyle	Continuum technique
	Ache deep in joint	Frogleg or reverse frogleg tectonic technique with compression force directed into elbow
	Elbow tightness with diminished internal rotation of shoulder	Indian burn cylinder technique
	Elbow feels stiff	Frogleg or reverse frogleg tectonic technique
Forearm Pain	Sweeping motion with fingers up and down forearm	Triggerband technique
	Points with one finger to source of pain	Continuum technique
	Pushes thumb deep into anterior forearm or grasps tightly with fingers and tugs on radius or ulna	Folding technique of interosseous membrane
Carpal Tunnel Syndrome	Tingling or *pins and needles* in median nerve distribution	Double thumb cylinder technique of flexor retinaculum
	Tingling or *pins and needles* throughout entire hand, wrist, and/or forearm	Indian burn cylinder technique of forearm followed by double thumb cylinder technique of retinaculum
	Tingling or *pins and needles* from shoulder down arm to wrist or hand	Squeegee cylinder technique of upper arm, Indian burn cylinder technique of forearm and wrist

Condition	Body Language/ Description of Discomfort	Orthopathic Treatment
Hand Pain	Pushes thumb into thenar eminence	Triggerband technique
	Pushes thumb onto metacarpal and locates spot(s) of pain	Continuum technique
	Diffuse pain deep in hand	Folding technique
	Boxer's fracture	Folding technique followed by continuum technique
Finger Pain	Fracture: Spiral	Triggerband technique
	Chip	Continuum technique
	Comminuted	Folding technique
	Pain deep in interphalangeal joint	Folding technique
	Stubbed fingers	Refolding followed by unfolding technique
	Osteoarthritis of fingers	Folding technique followed by continuum technique
	Diffuse finger pain	Indian burn cylinder technique
	Stiff fingers	Tectonic technique
Neck Pain	Sweeping motion with fingers along posterior neck	Triggerband technique of star triggerband
	Sweeping motion with fingers along lateral neck	Triggerband technique of upper trapezius (shoulder to mastoid) triggerband
	Wry neck	Triggerband technique of sternocleidomastoid muscle

Condition	Body Language/ Description of Discomfort	Orthopathic Treatment
Neck Pain	Aching at base of neck or pushes on supraclavicular fossa	Herniated triggerpoint therapy of SCHTP
	Spot(s) of pain	Continuum technique and/or thrusting manipulation
	Pain behind ear/points with finger to rim of atlas	Continuum technique or thrusting manipulation of atlas
	Ache deep in neck, pain lessened with traction	Unfolding technique (i.e., traction/thrust)
	Ache deep in neck, pain increased with traction	Refolding technique (i.e., compression/thrust)
	Squeezes neck	Double thumb cylinder technique
	Tingling	Double thumb cylinder technique
	Stiffness	Neutral thrust manipulation
Upper Back Pain	Sweeping motion with fingers from transverse process of T6 up to neck or mastoid	Triggerband technique of star
	Sweeping motion with fingers along upper trapezius muscle	Triggerband technique of shoulder to mastoid pathway
	Pushes with fingers into supraclavicular fossa	Herniated triggerpoint therapy of SCHTP
	Hurts in spot(s)	Continuum technique and/or neutral thrust
	Motor vehicle accident – aches deep in spine	Chair technique with traction or compression
	Reaches over shoulder and tugs up on mid-posterior ribs with fingers	Star folding manipulation

Condition	Body Language/ Description of Discomfort	Orthopathic Treatment
Upper Back Pain	Tugs or pulls on spinous process of upper thoracic vertebrae	Hallelujah maneuver
	Ache deep in lower thoracic spine	Wall technique (unfolding) chair technique (unfolding or refolding)
	First rib tightness	Swimmers position for 1st rib refolding thrust
	Ache deep in spine, feels worse with stretching	Turtle position or chair technique with compression
	Hurts with traction or compression	Inversion therapy (combination unfolding and refolding therapy)
	Stiffness	Kirksville crunch (dog technique) or chair neutral thrust
Fibromyalgia		Treatment Steps: 1. SCHTP, then triggerbands: star, upper trapezius, posterior shoulder pathway, consider comb technique 2. Folding distortions: first rib (refolding), star, paravertebral (chair and wall techniques, hallelujah maneuver, and inversion therapy) 3. Tectonic fixations: shoulder (frogleg and reverse frogleg manipulations), cervical (neutral thrust), thoracic (Kirksville crunch and chair technique with neutral thrust), low back (lumbar roll or chair neutral thrust) 4. Continuum distortions: continuum technique to affected areas 5. Cylinder distortions: squeegee technique for broad areas, double thumb for isolated spots, and Indian burn for forearm

Condition	Body Language/ Description of Discomfort	Orthopathic Treatment
Chest Wall Pain	Short sweeping strokes with fingers	Triggerband technique
	Points with one finger to source of pain	Continuum technique
	Tightness between ribs	Folding technique
Flank Pain	Sweeping motion with fingers from flank to groin	Triggerband technique of flank triggerband
	Pushes thumb into flank	Herniated triggerpoint therapy of flank HTP
Abdominal Pain	Presses fingers into abdomen and makes slow, sweeping strokes along a short linear pathway	Deep triggerband technique
	Pushes thumb into abdomen	Deep herniated triggerpoint therapy
Low Back Pain	Sweeping motion of fingers up and down posterior thigh	Triggerband technique of low back pain with thigh tightness triggerband
	Sweeping motion of fingers up and down iliotibial band	Triggerband technique of lateral thigh triggerband
	Pushes thumb forcefully into gluteal muscle	Herniated triggerpoint therapy of gluteal bull's-eye
	Points with one finger to PSIS	Continuum technique followed by thrusting manipulation (scissors technique)
	Back of hand or fist over lumbar vertebrae	Chair technique –traction/thrust (unfolding) or compression/thrust (refolding)
	Squeezes low back muscles with hands or fingers	Double thumb cylinder technique
	Stiffness	Chair neutral thrust

Condition	Body Language/ Description of Discomfort	Orthopathic Treatment
Low Back Pain	Places hands over iliac crest	Frogleg and reverse frogleg tectonic techniques of hip
Hip Pain	Sweeping motion with fingers along: 1. lateral thigh 2. mid-gluteus, 3. sacrum, or 4. iliac crest	Triggerband technique
	Pushes fingers or knuckles into mid-lateral gluteus maximus (bull's-eye)	Herniated triggerpoint therapy followed by continuum technique (if necessary)
	Points with one finger into sacroiliac joint	Continuum technique followed by scissors technique
	Ache deep in hip	Unfolding technique – traction/thrust
	Ache deep in hip and pushes fingers across anterior femoral head	Refolding technique – compression/thrust
	Places hands over iliac crests	Frogleg and reverse frogleg tectonic techniques
Thigh Pain	Pulled muscle	Triggerband technique
	Pulling or burning on posterior aspect	Triggerband technique of low back pain with thigh tightness triggerband
	Sweeping motion with fingers over lateral thigh	Triggerband technique of lateral thigh triggerband
	Diffuse discomfort, aching, or tingling	Indian burn cylinder technique
	Squeezes or pinches small portion of thigh	Double thumb cylinder technique
	Sweeping motion with palm or entire hand over broad area of anterior or lateral aspect of thigh	Squeegee cylinder technique

Condition	Body Language/ Description of Discomfort	Orthopathic Treatment
Knee Pain	Two inch sweeping motion with fingers from superior patella upwards	Triggerband technique
	Pushes fingers into popliteal fossa	Continuum or triggerband technique
	Point of pain, medial aspect	Continuum technique
	Osgood-Schlatter disease	Continuum technique
	Ache deep in joint, gently cups knee with hand, tugs on thigh	Unfolding technique
	Ache deep in joint, cups knee with hand and rubs fingers back and forth across inferior knee	Refolding technique
	Diffuse pain	Indian burn cylinder technique
	Small area of vague discomfort, exact location cannot be determined	Double thumb cylinder technique
	Feels like it needs to pop	Frogleg and reverse frogleg tectonic techniques
Leg Pain	Shin splints, pain along anterior leg	Triggerband technique
	Shin splints, pain in spots	Continuum technique
	Deep ache in leg	Folding technique of interosseous membrane
	Diffuse pain over entire leg, repetitively squeezes several portions of leg	Indian burn cylinder technique
	Tourniquet sensation	Squeegee cylinder technique

Condition	Body Language/ Description of Discomfort	Orthopathic Treatment
Ankle Sprain	Pulling pain up calf	Triggerband technique
	Pain in one or more spots	Continuum technique
	Pain deep in joint, grasps ankle with hand, prominent bi-malleolar swelling	Traction/thrust (unfolding)
	Pain deep in joint, grasps ankle with hand then rubs finger across ankle	Compression/thrust (refolding)
	Pain diffusely on dorsal aspect of ankle	Double thumb cylinder technique
	Long-standing ankle stiffness	Frogleg and reverse frogleg tectonic techniques
Foot Sprain	Pain along linear pathway	Triggerband technique
	Point tenderness	Continuum technique
	Swelling/ache deep in foot between metatarsal bones	Folding technique
	Pain diffusely on dorsal aspect of foot with or without swelling, unable to localize area of discomfort	Double thumb cylinder technique
	Long-standing foot stiffness	Tectonic technique
Foot fracture	Pain in spot(s) with generalized aching	Gentle folding technique followed by continuum technique
Plantar Fasciitis	Sweeping motion with fingers along bottom of foot	Triggerband technique
	Points to spot(s) of pain on calcaneus	Continuum technique

Condition	Body Language/ Description of Discomfort	Orthopathic Treatment
Toe Sprain	Pain along length of toe	Triggerband technique
	Spot of pain	Continuum technique
	Ache with swelling	Unfolding technique
	Stubbed toes	Refolding followed by unfolding technique
	Diffuse pain	Indian burn cylinder technique
Toe fracture		Gentle folding technique followed by continuum technique

Treatment of Combination Distortions

Chronic pain – Treat triggerbands with adhesions first, then correct acute injury

Triggerbands & HTP's (a.k.a. banded HTP) – Treat HTP first

Triggerbands & Continuum Distortions – Correct triggerbands first

Triggerbands & Folding – Treat triggerbands first

Triggerbands & Tectonic Fixations – Treat triggerbands first

HTP's and any of the following –
    Continuum Distortions
    Folding Distortions
    Cylinder Distortions
    Tectonic Fixations   – Treat HTP first

Continuum Distortions & Folding Distortions – Generally treat CD first
    If everted, wait 24 hours to treat folding distortion

Continuum Distortions & Cylinders – Treat continuum distortions first

Continuum Distortions & Tectonic Fixations – Treat TF first

Refolding & Unfolding – Refold first then unfold

Cylinders & Tectonic Fixations – Correct cylinders first *and* last

Cylinders and other distortions – Correct cylinders last

Tectonic Fixation & Refolding – Correct folding distortion first

Multiple Combinations – Treat in this order
1. HTP
2. Triggerbands
3. Tectonic Fixations
4. Folding Distortions
5. Continuum Distortions
6. Cylinder Distortions

ORTHOPATHIC ABBREVIATIONS

AACD	Anterior Ankle Continuum Distortion
CCV	Compression Cylinder Variant
CD	Continuum Distortion
CT	Continuum Technique
CTS	Carpal Tunnel Syndrome (or Carpal Tunnel Symptoms)
CyD	Cylinder Distortion
CyT	Cylinder Technique
ECD	Everted Continuum Distortion
FD	Folding Distortion
FDM	Fascial Distortion Model
FDT	Fascial Distortion Technique
FT	Folding Technique
HTP	Herniated Triggerpoint
HTPT	Herniated Triggerpoint Therapy
HVLA	High-Velocity Low-Amplitude osteopathic manipulation
ICD	Inverted Continuum Distortion
LBP	Low Back Pain
OM	Orthopathic Medicine
PSSP	Post-Stroke Spastic Paralysis
PSSPP	Post-Stroke Spastic Paralysis Patient
RFD	Refolding Distortion
RFT	Refolding Technique
SCHTP	Supraclavicular Herniated Triggerpoint
SI	Sacroiliac joint
SP	Starting Point
TB	Triggerband
TBT	Triggerband Technique
TF	Tectonic Fixation
TMJ	Temporomandibular Joint
TT	Tectonic Technique
TZ	Transition Zone
UFD	Unfolding Distortion
UFT	Unfolding Technique

Comparison of Principal

Comparative Category	Etiology	Picture	Subtypes
Triggerband	Distorted fascial bands		1. Twist 2. Crumple 3. Knot 4. Pea 5. Grain of salt 6. Wave
Herniated Triggerpoint	Protrusion of tissue through fascial plane		1. Non-banded 2. Banded
Continuum Distortion	Alteration of transition zone between tissue types		1. Everted 2. Inverted
Folding Distortion	Three dimensional alteration of fascial plane		1. Unfolding 2. Refolding
Cylinder Distortion	Tangling of circular fascia		1. Superficial 2. Deep
Tectonic Fixation	Loss of ability of fascial surface to glide		None currently recognized

Types of Fascial Distortions

Movement During Treatment	Common Locations	Common Injuries Associated with Distortion	Most Specific Treatment
Yes, linear	Throughout the body along well demarcated pathways	Ankle sprains, sore shoulders, tendonitis, whiplash injuries, pulled muscles, many other acute and all chronic injuries	Triggerband Technique
Non-banded=no Banded=yes	Supraclavicular fossa, abdomen, flank, buttock	Sore shoulders, neck pain, abdominal pain, renal colic pain	Herniated Triggerpoint Therapy
No	Origin or insertion of tendon or ligament with bone	Ankle sprains, sore shoulders, wrist sprains, rib fractures, sacroiliac pain, foot sprains, contusions	Continuum Technique
No	Interosseous membranes, spine, and joints	Ankle sprains, sore shoulders, foot sprains, finger sprains, fractures, dislocations, back pain	Folding Technique
No, but jumping phenomenon is common	Extremities and trunk	Sore shoulders (upper arm pain), low back spasm, carpal tunnel syndrome, foot sprains	Cylinder Technique
No	Shoulder, hip, elbow, knee, facet joints	Frozen shoulder (adhesive capsulitis), stiff low back	Tectonic Technique

Triggerband Subtypes

Subtype	Palpatory Sensation	Palpatory Dimension	Common Locations
Twist	Twisted ribbon edge	Suture to pencil width	Throughout the body
Crumple	Tingling sensation	1/8" to 1/4" wide	Between muscle layers
Knot	Knotted-up rubber band	Almond shape	Thoracic and lumbar areas
Pea	Cooked pea	Pea size	Neck, thighs, upper arms
Grain of Salt	Firm with irregular edges (scraping sensation)	Salt grain size	Face, scalp, hands, feet
Wave	Wrinkling of tissue	Barely palpable	Near joints

Note that triggerband subtypes represent the clinical spectrum of triggerband palpatory findings. Peas are in essence a smaller and softer version of a knot, and crumples are larger forms of waves. As the triggerband is corrected with triggerband technique, the distorted fascial band may present along its course as several different subtypes. For instance, the star triggerband in the thoracic area typically is palpated as a knot. But during treatment as it passes through the neck, it may feel like a pea. And the same distortion just a few seconds later when it is traced under the occiput or onto the mastoid process palpates as a twist or even a grain of salt.

Herniated Triggerpoint Subtypes

Subtype	Etiology	Palpatory Presentation	Treatment
Non-banded	Protrusion of tissue through a non-banded fascial plane	Soft, almond-sized (or smaller) elevation in tissue	Herniated triggerpoint therapy (i.e., the protruding tissue is forced below the fascial plane with pressure from the physician's thumb)
Banded	Protrusion of tissue through a fascial plane distorted by a triggerband	Same as above except that at the completion of herniated triggerpoint therapy a triggerband is palpated	Herniated triggerpoint therapy followed by triggerband technique

Continuum Distortion Subtypes

Comparative Category	Everted	Inverted
Etiology	Portion of transition zone between ligament or tendon and bone stuck in *osseous* configuration	Portion of transition zone between ligament or tendon and bone stuck in *ligamentous* configuration
Size	*O* to *o*	*O* to *o*
Palpatory Sensation Analogy	Vitamin A or E soft-gel capsule, or the edge of the eraser on end of pencil	Hole in trouser belt that buckle prong pierces
Most Specific Treatment	Continuum technique	Continuum technique and HVLA
Common Injuries	Ankle sprains, fractured ribs, wrist sprains	Sacroiliac strains, bony contusions, whiplash injuries

Folding Distortion Subtypes

Comparative Category	Unfolding	Refolding
Mechanism Of Injury	Limb/vertebrae pulled or jerked away from joint (traction force)	Limb/vertebrae pushed or shoved into joint (compression force)
Pathology	Folding fascia stuck in the partially unfolded position	Folding fascia stuck in the partially refolded position
Structural Ramification	Folding fascia can't refold completely	Folding fascia can't unfold completely
What Makes It Hurt	Pushing limb/vertebra into joint (compression)	Traction of limb/vertebrae away from joint (traction)
What Makes It Feel Better	Traction (pulling)	Compression (pushing)
Treatment	Unfolding technique (pulling or thrusting limb/vertebrae away from joint, i.e., traction)	Refolding technique (pushing or thrusting limb/vertebrae into joint, i.e., compression)

Cylinder Distortion Subtypes

Subtype	Etiology	Palpatory Presentation	Most Specific Treatment
Deep	Tangled coils of less superficial layer of cylinder fascia	Taut tissue	Double thumb cylinder technique with traction *perpendicular* to axis of bones
Superficial	Tangled coils of most superficial layer of cylinder fascia	Taut tissue	Double thumb cylinder technique with traction *parallel* to axis of bones

GLOSSARY

Abduction: Shoulder motion in which the hands are brought from the sides of the body up and over the head with the elbows extended.

Acupuncture Points: Specific anatomical sites in which acupuncture needles are placed. These commonly match crossbands of triggerbands, and the acupuncture meridians often correspond to triggerband pathways.

Acute Injury: Musculoskeletal dysfunction in which no adhesions have formed.

Adhesions: Fascial fibers (torn crosslinks) that aberrantly attach to other structures and result in dysfunction and restriction of those structures.

Adhesive Capsulitis: A severe form of tectonic fixation that is compounded with triggerbands and fascial adhesions.

Allopathic Medicine: Dominant form of medicine practiced in the United States. Graduates of these medical schools are designated as Doctor of Medicine and use the abbreviation M.D. Historically, allopaths treat diseases by producing a condition incompatible or antagonistic to the condition treated (basis of most current pharmaceutical therapies such as aspirin which is antagonistic to fever). In contrast to allopathy is *homeopathy* which prescribes minute doses of a substance to produce symptoms similar to the condition treated (basis of immunizations).

All-or-None Principle: Clinical phenomena that occurs during continuum technique in which either the transition zone shifts or it doesn't. Because of the all-or-none principle, a partial resolution is not possible with continuum technique.

Aneurysm: Herniated triggerpoint of blood vessel.

Angina: Temporary ischemic changes in the heart, perhaps brought on by a distorted fascial band constricting a coronary artery.

Ankle Eversion: Motion in which the ankle buckles laterally.

Ankle Sprain: Soft tissue injury to the ankle in which there is swelling, pain, and loss of motion, but no fracture. In the FDM, ankle sprains occur in three varieties: continuum, triggerband, and folding.

Anterior Ankle Continuum Distortion: Continuum distortion present on the anterior aspect of every ankle sprain of every type. It is primarily responsible for loss of foot dorsiflexion.

Anterior Shoulder Triggerband Pathway: Course of the triggerband responsible for bicipital tendonitis, and pain and tightness in the front of the shoulder. Its starting point is on the proximal anterior forearm and its pathway courses superiorly through the bicipital groove up to the ipsilateral mastoid process.

Arteriosclerosis: Narrowing of the blood vessel with plaque formation, perhaps secondary to a fascial distortion on the exterior of the vessel constricting the lumen.

Asthma: Sudden onset of bronchiole constriction which could be secondary to a simultaneous tightening of all the fascial bands in the lung (see *Purse String Effect*).

Babst Board: Flat board with half-spheres beneath which is used by physical therapists as a form of teeter-totter to increase proprioception following an ankle sprain. In the FDM, rocking back and forth on the board gently untwists twisted fascial fibers in the ankle, leg, and thigh, thus restoring the normal ability of those fibers to function as an accessory mechanical sensory system. The rocking motion also unfolds and refolds the ankle capsule helping to correct folding distortions.

Ball Therapy: Therapy balls of assorted sizes and shapes are used in conjunction with both folding and tectonic techniques. The involved joint is placed over the ball during the treatment and either a thrusting manipulation (tectonic technique), traction (unfolding technique), or compression (refolding technique) is initiated. During thrusting manipulation the ball indents and recoils which lubricates the joint at the moment of the thrust by pumping fluid directly between the fixated surfaces. In folding technique, the ball supports the joint comfortably in a wide variety of positions so that traction or compression can be focused into the restricted areas.

Banded Herniated Triggerpoint: Subtype of herniated triggerpoint characterized by protrusion of tissue through a banded fascial plane that is distorted by a triggerband.

Banded Pseudo-Triggerpoint: Fascial distortion that occurs when two or more triggerbands overlap (common in fibromyalgia).

Behind-the-Eye Headache: Typical description of symptoms caused by a combination distortion of a triggerband and a lacrimal herniated triggerpoint.

Biliary Colic: Narrowing of the bile duct from either a triggerband or a herniated triggerpoint which results in spasm as a stone attempts to pass.

Body Language: Consistent subconscious motions or postures exhibited by patients with specific fascial distortions.

Brute Force Maneuver of the Scapula: Tectonic technique in which the palm of the treating hand is used to induce the scapula to slide.

Brute Force Maneuver of the Shoulder: Tectonic technique in which the weight of the physician is used to induce the capsule to slide. This is accomplished by having the physician transfer his/her weight onto the patient's shoulders through his/her hands. Note that the doctor stands behind the patient and his/her right palm is positioned on the patient's right shoulder and the doctor's left palm is placed on the patient's left shoulder (an accompanying rocking motion pumps synovial fluid and helps budge the capsule).

Bull's-Eye Herniated Triggerpoint: HTP of the gluteal area. It is often accompanied by a continuum distortion directly beneath it.

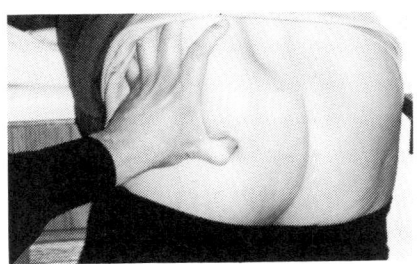

Bursitis: Painful area under a muscle that is tender to touch. Clinically most are either triggerbands or continuum distortions.

Button Slipping Into the Buttonhole Analogy: Sensation of both patient and physician at the moment of correction of a continuum distortion.

Cable Ligaments: Huge fascial bands along the vertebrae of certain dinosaurs.

Carpal Tunnel Syndrome: Fascial distortions of the wrist retinaculum and fascia that result in symptoms of burning, numbness, tingling, or pain in the wrist, forearm, fingers, or hand. Cylinder distortions and triggerbands are the most common etiologies.

Chair Technique: Sitting folding/thrusting manipulation of the lumbar and thoracic spine. In the FDM when the thrust is accompanied with traction it is an unfolding technique and when the thrust is accompanied with compression it becomes a refolding technique. Note: A neutral thrust manipulation (no traction or compression) is utilized to treat facet tectonic fixations and inverted continuum distortions.

Chronic Injury: Musculoskeletal dysfunction in which fascial adhesions have formed.

Comb Technique: Therapy in which a metal comb is raked across the skin to fracture fascial adhesions and to untangle cylinder fascia.

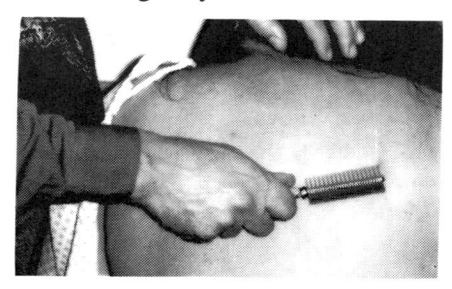

Combination Distortion: Injury comprised of two or more principal fascial distortion types (such as a continuum distortion and a triggerband).

Combination Sprained Ankle: Sprained ankle that clinically presents with two or three principal fascial distortion types.

Compression Cylinder Variant: Modification of cylinder technique (Indian burn, double thumb, and squeegee) in which the fascial coils are pushed together rather than pulled apart.

Compression/Thrust: Manipulation in which a sustained pushing force is combined with a rapid pushing or rotational force (HVLA) to refold folding fascia.

Continuity Model of Anatomy: Anatomical perspective in which individual fascial fibers pass through other tissues and link all of those tissues together into a single structural unit. Any alteration of the fiber anywhere along its path is thought to cause dysfunction in every portion of that pathway. In addition, the fascial fibers are considered to be continuous with and become the fibers that make up bone, ligaments, and other connective tissues.

Continuum Distortion: Principal fascial distortion type that occurs when there is an alteration of the transition zone between two tissue types. This most commonly occurs at the origin or insertion of ligaments or tendons with bone.

Continuum Model of Anatomy: Anatomical perspective in which tissue types are viewed as being a continuum of each other. Depending on the intrinsic and extrinsic forces applied, tissues may take on characteristics of adjoining tissues through their common transition zone.

Continuum Technique: Manual modality to treat continuum distortions. Force is applied by the physician's thumb directly into the area of shifted continuum. It is held until the transition zone is forced to shift (i.e., release).

Contusion (bony): Continuum distortion of the periosteum.

Contusion (muscle): Cylinder distortion of superficial fascia overlying the affected muscle.

Cornstarch/Water Phenomenon: Simple laboratory demonstration in which cornstarch is mixed with water to show that the physical properties of this amorphous substance are determined by the external forces introduced into it. When stirred (i.e., forces from more than one direction are introduced at the same time) the cornstarch/water compound acts as a liquid, but when poked or tapped (i.e., force is directed into it from only one direction) it behaves as a solid. The transition zone between bone and ligament is thought to have a similar ability in that it is capable of instantaneously shifting back and forth between osseous and ligamental configurations depending on the external forces encountered.

Cortisone Injection of Joint: In the FDM the injected solution increases the volume of liquid in the joint and flushes stagnant synovial fluid out of the joint.

Cows Through the Barn Door Analogy: Comparison made between herding cows into the barn and correcting herniated triggerpoints.

Costochondritis: Chest wall pain resulting from a combination of triggerbands and continuum distortions.

Cranial Technique: Treatment modality in which the rhythm of fascial fluid is palpated in the cranial area and gentle alterations of the rhythm are made to influence fascial distortions at a distant site.

Crisscrossing Fascial Bands: Potential site for two triggerband twists to meet and become locked in place.

Crossband: Fascial band found in the same plane and at a different angle to a triggerband. Crossbands are often the anatomical starting place for triggerband technique.

Crosslink: Single perpendicular fiber of a fascial band that holds the parallel fibers of the band together. When the crosslink is torn, the fascial fibers are then able to twist, separate and tear apart. When the injured crosslinks pathologically reattach to inappropriate structures (such as other fascial bands) they are called fascial adhesions.

Crumple: Distorted fascial band wedged between muscle layers – a triggerband subtype.

Cupping: Method of treating tectonic fixations in which glass or plastic cups are suctioned onto the skin overlying joints.

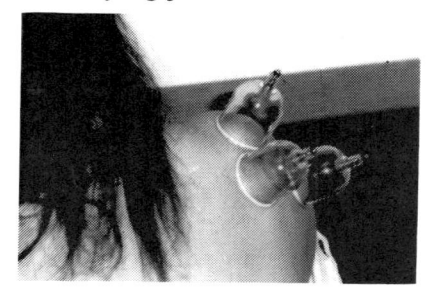

Cylinder Distortion: Principal type of fascial distortion characterized as an alteration of circular fascia in which the cylindric coils have become tangled.

Cylinder Fascia: Superficial fascia that encircles the extremities. (Note that cylinder fascia may also occur in other areas of the body such as the trunk, thorax, and blood vessels, including the coronary arteries).

Cylinder Shuffle: Characteristic gait associated with cylinder distortions of the lower leg.

Cylinder Technique: Manual therapy designed to correct cylinder distortions. Five cylinder techniques currently in use: 1. Indian burn, 2. double thumb, 3. comb for chronic cylinder distortions, 4. squeegee, and 5. compression cylinder variants.

Double Thumb Cylinder Technique: Manual method for correcting cylinder distortions in which the overlapped and tangled cylindric fascial coils are tractioned apart by the treating doctor's thumbs.

Double Twist: Triggerband distortion in which the fascial band is twisted twice. These are thought to be the cause of the headlight effect.

Everted Continuum Distortion: Subtype of continuum distortion in which a portion of the transition zone is stuck in the osseous configuration.

External Rotation: Shoulder motion in which the hands are placed behind the neck and the fingers are intertwined. The elbows are then pushed posteriorly.

Fascia: Primary connective tissue of the body that makes up tendons, ligaments, fascial bands, myofascia, adhesions, retinacula, and other tissues that surround and engulf muscles, bones, nerves, and organs.

Fascial Band: Collection of parallel fascial fibers.

Fascial Distortion: Pathological alteration of fascia that results in dysfunction of the affected fascia and its associated structures.

Fascial Distortion Model: Anatomical perspective in which musculoskeletal injuries are envisioned as consisting of specific alterations in the body's fascia (see *Principal Types of Fascial Distortions*). As a model, the FDM is an abbreviated interpretation of the pathology of fascial injuries and contemplates the structural consequences of osteopathic and orthopedic interventions.

Fascial Fiber: Collection of parallel collagen fibers.

Fascial Plane: Fascial tissue that is broad and wide but has little thickness.

Fasciitis: 1. Infection of fascia, 2. a non-specific term used to describe a fascial distortion (example: plantar fasciitis).

Fibromyalgia: Multiple fascial distortions involving large areas of the body with excessive fascial adhesion formation.

Flank Herniated Triggerpoint: HTP associated with renal colic.

Flank Triggerband: Triggerband associated with renal colic.

Flaring: Amount of space between elbow and body during internal rotation of the shoulder.

Fluidity: Smoothness of motion.

Folding Distortion: Principal fascial distortion type that is the result of a three-dimensional alteration of the fascial plane.

Folding Fascia: Fascia that has the ability to unfold during stress and refold when the stress is removed.

Folding/High-Velocity Manipulation: a.k.a. folding/thrusting manipulation, two kinds: 1. Combination of traction, which unfolds the fascia, and pulling-thrusting manipulation (traction/thrust unfolding technique), and 2. Combination of compression, which refolds the fascia, and pushing-thrusting manipulation (compression/thrust refolding technique).

Folding Technique: Modified traction approach which is designed to unfold distorted folding fascia and allow it to refold properly, or modified compression approach which refolds distorted folding fascia and allows it to unfold properly.

Foot Inversion: Motion in which the ankle buckles laterally.

Foot Sprain: Injury to the soft tissue of the foot that involves continuum distortions, cylinder distortions, triggerbands, and/or folding distortions.

Forearm Cross: Technique for correcting a shoulder capsule tectonic fixation.

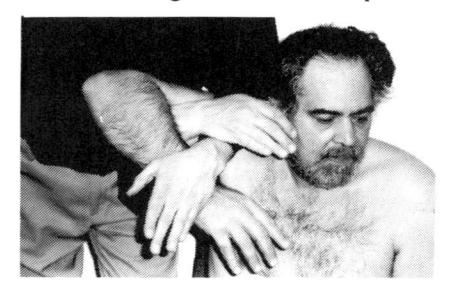

Fracture: Extension of fascial distortions into the osseous matrix.

Frogleg Tectonic Manipulations of the Hip and Shoulder: Treatment to correct tectonic fixations of either the femur in the acetabulum or the humerus in the glenoid fossa. In these procedures the affected limb is placed into an extreme Patrick-Fabere position and a thrust is made. When the frogleg manipulation is performed in the reverse Patrick-Fabere position it is called *reverse frogleg tectonic technique*. In addition to correcting tectonic fixations of the hip and shoulder, frogleg and reverse frogleg manipulations can be modified to correct tectonic fixations of the elbow, knee, and ankle. Note: "F-ab-er-e" is a mnemonic formula ("F" for flexion, "ab" for abduction, "er" for external rotation, and "e" for extension).

Frozen Shoulder: Any shoulder exhibiting reduction or loss of abduction, external rotation, internal rotation, or other motions.

Global Loss of Motion: Impairment in all three primary shoulder motions – abduction, external rotation, and internal rotation.

John Godman: Nineteenth century American physician and anatomist who stressed the importance of understanding fascia.

Grain of Salt: Triggerband subtype that is very small with irregular edges.

Groin Pull: Triggerband present in the groin.

Hallelujah Maneuver: Lifting/unfolding manipulation of the upper thoracic spine that is performed either sitting or standing. Note that by simultaneously applying torque to the shoulder, the forces can be directed into the gleno-humeral joint.

Hand Direction: Orientation of hand during internal rotation of the shoulder. Vertical direction (i.e., the fingers are pointing up) is optimal.

Hand Rotation: Ability to place the palm flat against the back during internal rotation of the shoulder.

Headlight Effect: The patient's awareness of the course of the triggerband pathway some distance ahead of the actual point of the triggerband treatment. The cause of this is thought to be a double twist in the fascial band (the second twist is pushed ahead by pressure being applied to the first twist).

Heel Spur Continuum Distortion: Continuum distortion palpated at the junction of the plantar fascia and calcaneus that together with a triggerband is responsible for plantar fasciitis.

Herniated Triggerpoint: Principal fascial distortion type that results from tissue protruding through a fascial plane.

Herniated Triggerpoint Therapy: Technique used to correct herniated triggerpoints in which the physician's thumb pushes the protruding tissue below the fascial plane.

Hesitation: Decrease in speed of extremity during a portion of its motion.

High-Velocity Low-Amplitude Osteopathic Manipulation (HVLA): Vertebrae or other bones are forcefully manipulated so that the joint surfaces suddenly move. When this occurs an articular sound is audible. HVLA is useful in treating many injuries. It can sling-shot a small triggerband twist away from a joint or direct a pulling force directly into an inverted continuum distortion. When HVLA is combined with traction or compression it can correct folding distortions. In addition, HVLA can break tectonic fixations by directing a "sliding" force into joint capsules and facet joints. Because of these potential benefits, HVLA is a useful tool in the treatment of tectonic fixations and simple acute injuries secondary to a triggerband, inverted continuum or folding distortion. In chronic injuries HVLA is rarely successful until after the fascial adhesions have been fractured by either triggerband technique or comb technique.

Hit-By-Truck Effect: Dramatic subjective increase in the symptoms of a chronic pain patient following the first one or two triggerband technique treatments.

Hypertonicity: Increased muscle tone as the result of continuous electrical stimulation.

Ice/Slush/Water Analogy: Comparison of how external physical forces determine both the stages of water and the configurations of the transition zone between ligament or tendon and bone.

Indian Burn Cylinder Technique: Cylinder technique in which traction is maintained with both hands as rotation is applied so that one hand torques in a clockwise direction while the other hand does so in a counterclockwise direction. This technique should be avoided in the upper arm, foot, and ankle.

Integrated Neuromusculoskeletal Release: (INR) Isometric-isotonic, functional, and myofascial release techniques combined with patient-assisted maneuvers such as breath-holding, motion of the extremities, changes in body position, or cranial nerve activities such as eye, tongue, or jaw movement. Cylinder and folding distortions may respond to this therapy.

Internal Rotation: Shoulder motion in which the back of the hand can be placed against the back of the body.

Inversion Therapy: Correction of folding distortions of the spine with either ball therapy or inversion traction. In either case, the patient is placed in a retracted but supported position and, with assistance from the physical therapist, uses his/her own weight and movement to elongate (and thus unfold) or compress (and refold) the paravertebral fascia.

Inverted Continuum Distortion: Subtype of continuum distortion in which a portion of the transition zone is stuck in the ligamental configuration.

Jumping Phenomenon: Non-contiguous change of location of pain as the result of treatment with cylinder technique.

Karate-Chop Hand Arrangement: One possible hand position taken when treating a tectonic fixation of the shoulder capsule.

Key Bronchus Triggerband: Hypothetical triggerband that may be the initiator of the purse string effect.

Knot: Triggerband subtype that occurs when a portion of a fascial band has been ripped from its attachment and has knotted upon itself.

Lacrimal Herniated Triggerpoint: HTP near the lacrimal bone associated with behind-the-eye headaches.

Lateral Ankle Triggerband Pathway: Most common pathway present in a triggerband sprained ankle. It originates on the lateral ankle at the sock line and in treating with triggerband technique, it is followed inferiorly to behind the lateral malleolus and then along the lateral dorsal foot to the base of a toe (fourth and fifth are most common).

Lateral Recumbent Folding Technique of the Shoulder: Unfolding technique in which the patient is laid on the side (affected shoulder up) and traction/thrust is introduced into the shoulder with direction of force toward the elbow.

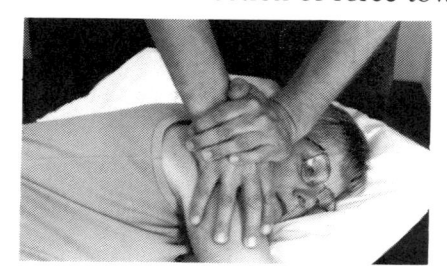

Linea Coli: Large fascial band present on colon.

Loaded Ligamental Fibers: Uninjured ligamental fibers that straighten with extrinsic force.

Low Back Pain with Thigh Tightness Triggerband: Triggerband that originates in the posterior thigh and courses superiorly over the buttock to the low back and then inferiorly to the sacrococcygeal junction. It is a common cause of low back, sacroiliac, and thigh pain.

Lunging: Slight increase in the speed of motion of an extremity following hesitation.

Massage: Treatment of myofascia that moves small triggerbands away from the muscle. Massage may also help straighten ruffled cylinder fascia and break fascial adhesions.

McBurney's Point: Almond-sized tender area in right lower quadrant of abdomen that typically is associated with an acute appendicitis. In the FDM, McBurney's point is anatomically a herniated triggerpoint which forms from the inflammation forcing adjacent tissue through the neighboring fascial plane.

Milking a Release: In herniated triggerpoint therapy and continuum technique, the thumb is gently rocked back and forth during the releasing process.

Movement: Motion of a triggerband twist along its pathway during triggerband technique.

Muscle Energy Technique: Treatment modality in which muscle contractions are used to force a triggerband twist out of a muscle.

Myocardial Infarction: In the FDM, coronary artery triggerbands and cylinder distortions are speculated to be responsible for some types of MI's.

Myofascial Release Technique: Treatment modality in which sustained manual traction is applied until a triggerband twist is pulled out of a muscle, a folding distortion is unfolded, or a cylinder distortion is untangled.

Myofascial Triggerpoint: See *Triggerpoint*.

Neutral Thrust: Purely rotational HVLA tectonic manipulation of a joint in which no traction or compression is utilized.

Non-banded Herniated Triggerpoint: Herniated triggerpoint subtype that is characterized as a protrusion of tissue through a non-banded fascial plane.

Orthopath: (a.k.a. orthopathist) Someone who practices orthopathy, i.e., physicians, international osteopaths, or surgeons who envision injuries through the fascial distortion model and whose treatment intent is to correct fascial distortions.

Orthopathic Medicine: (a.k.a. orthopathy) Broad term used to embrace the entire concept of unification of orthopedics with osteopathy through the fascial distortion model, its practice, and application. The term *orthopathy* is derived from the combination of the two words *ortho*pedics and osteo*pathy* and refers to the clinical manipulative practice of orthopathic medicine.

Orthopathic Medicine (archaic): (a.k.a. orthopathy) Theory of medicine (coincidentally with same name but unrelated to the theories, concepts, and techniques presented in this book) first made public by Issac Jennings, M.D. in 1822. This now-defunct branch of the healing arts stressed proper nutrition, avoidance of harmful drugs, and the recuperative powers of the body. In its heyday, it counted among its supporters auto industrialist Henry Ford, Dr. Graham of graham cracker fame, and Florence Nightingale (the founder of modern nursing). The last orthopathic medical school closed in 1908.

Orthopedics: Branch of surgery that focuses on the treatment of the skeletal system and associated structures.

Orthopedist: Orthopedic surgeon (either M.D. or D.O.). The term for an orthopedist who includes fascial distortion concepts into his/her surgical practice is *orthopathic surgeon*.

Osgood-Schlatter Disease: Continuum distortions of the tibial tuberosity.

Osteoarthritis: Condition in which distorted fascia in or near a joint has taken on characteristics of the adjoining bone.

Osteopath: One who practices osteopathy. In some countries osteopathic training focuses exclusively on osteopathy. In other countries, osteopathy is a form of advanced study for physicians and physical therapists. In the United States, osteopaths are graduates of four-year medical schools and have residency training in one or more of the dozens of fields of medicine such as orthopedics, general surgery, obstetrics, internal medicine, family practice, etc. These physicians are designated as Doctor of Osteopathy or Doctor of Osteopathic Medicine, and use the abbreviation D.O.

Osteopathic Medicine: Branch of the healing arts founded in 1874 by Andrew Taylor Still, M.D. that includes the full scope of medical and surgical practice integrated with osteopathic concepts.

Osteopathy: Manual practice of osteopathic medicine which stresses the interrelationship and importance of the musculoskeletal system in disease and injury. Practitioners of osteopathy employ a wide variety of manipulative techniques in the treatment of somatic dysfunction (palpatory restrictions, misalignments, or other anatomical abnormalities of the human structure).

Osteoporosis: Condition in which osseous components have either been drained out of the bone or have not been properly replenished or revitalized.

Overshift: Pathological condition of a portion of the transition zone between ligament or tendon and bone in which an excessive amount of osseous components have been transferred. If the overshift occurs from bone to ligament, this results in an everted continuum distortion. If the overshift occurs from ligament to bone, this results in an inverted continuum distortion.

Pea: Triggerband subtype that is smaller and smoother than a knot.

Percussion Hammer: Treatment in which a vibratory hammer delivers rapid, intermittent pressure into a restricted joint or tissue. Through the FDM this approach is envisioned as affecting tectonic fixations (pumping synovial fluid through the joint and coaxing the capsule to slide), triggerbands (pushing a twist out of the belly of a muscle or away from a joint), continuum distortions (forcing the transition zone to shift), cylinder distortions (stretching the fascial coils), and refolding distortions (over-folding misfolded fascia which then rebounds less contorted).

Pitch: Vibratory frequency of a fascial fiber.

Plantar Fasciitis: Triggerbands and/or continuum distortions of the plantar fascia.

Plunger Technique: Treatment utilizing suction to correct tectonic fixations by increasing circulation of stagnant synovial fluid. Shown below are standard sink plunger (left) and plunger hammer (right).

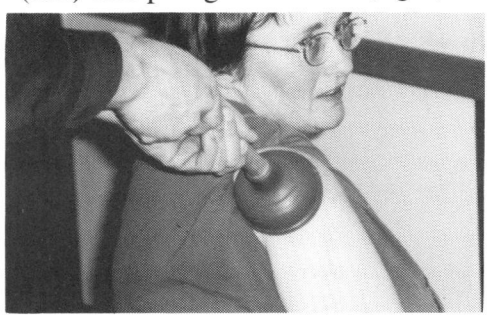

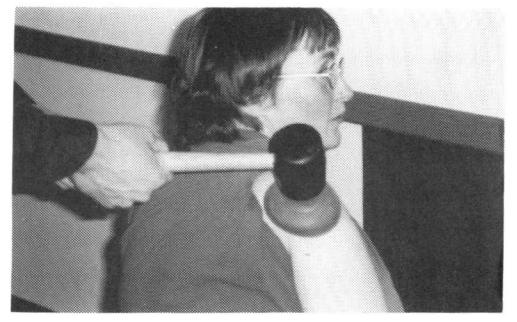

Posterior Shoulder Triggerband Pathway: Course of the triggerband responsible for posterior shoulder pain and tightness. Its starting point is on the posterior proximal forearm and it continues superiorly to the contralateral mastoid process.

Pressure Points: Small areas of the body that are tender to palpation. In the FDM, pressure points are non-differentiated fascial distortions (see *Triggerpoint*).

Principal Types of Fascial Distortions: Pathological alterations of fascia that have distinct etiologies. There are currently six described – triggerbands, herniated triggerpoints, continuum distortions, folding distortions, cylinder distortions, and tectonic fixations. For a new principal type to be recognized, it must have a completely different etiology than any of the principal distortion types previously described.

Prone Tectonic Technique of the Shoulder: Tectonic technique of the anterior shoulder capsule in which the patient is positioned prone and the elbow is flexed at a 90° angle. The correction is made by thrusting the forearm posteriorly while the upper arm is held against the table.

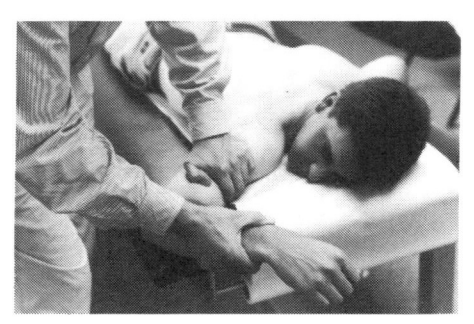

Pseudo-Sciatica: Any one of several triggerband pathways that mimic the course of the sciatic nerve.

Pulled Muscle: Distorted fascial band stuck in the belly of a muscle at an angle to the axis of the muscle.

Purse String Effect: Analogy to illustrate that in asthma all of the fascial fibers of the affected lung may become suddenly tightened from a single source.

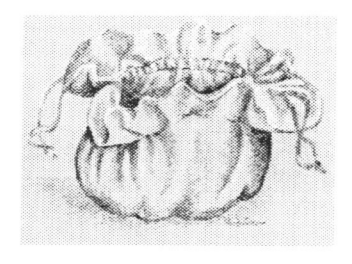

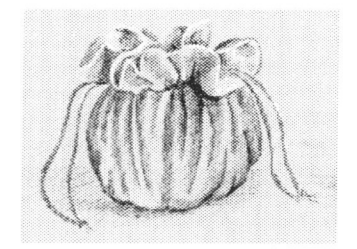

Quick Victory Strategy: Rapid correction of a fascial distortion to demonstrate objective efficacy of the treatment.

Refolding Distortion: Subtype of folding distortion in which fascia is over-compressed and can't unfold completely. Refolding injuries hurt deep in the joint, feel better with compression and worse with traction, and clinically respond to compression and/or compression/thrust manipulations (i.e., refolding techniques).

Release: Sensation experienced by both physician and patient at the instant of correction of a continuum distortion, herniated triggerpoint, folding distortion, or cylinder distortion. In HTP's the release feels like a melting and lasts from five up to fifteen seconds or more. The release of continuum technique is rapid (lasting only a few seconds) and to palpation is reminiscent of a button slipping into a buttonhole. Folding distortions release as a series of small clicks, and cylinder distortions have a very subtle release lasting only a few seconds that is perceived as a lessening in tissue tautness.

Renal Colic: Narrowing of the ureter secondary to a triggerband or herniated triggerpoint that results in spasm as a stone attempts to pass.

Road Map Analogy: Analogy comparing a common road map to folding fascia. Both are able to unfold and refold in the same manner, and both can become contorted if unfolded and twisted or over-compressed.

Rolfing: Manual treatment of fascia in which adhesions are broken.

Scissors Technique: Lateral recumbent manipulative approach utilized in the treatment of inverted continuum distortions of the sacroiliac joint. Note that by altering the direction of thrust the procedure can be modified to correct tectonic fixations and folding distortions of the SI joint, lumbar spine, sacral segments, and even the shoulder.

Sclerotherapy: In addition to facilitating adhesion formation, prolotherapy injections shift the transition zone from the neutral or ligamentous state into the osseous configuration. Thus, sclerotherapy can be envisioned as a chemical form of continuum technique.

Shifting of the Continuum: Ability of the transition zone between two different tissue types to change into a configuration of either type.

Shoulder to Mastoid Triggerband: (a.k.a. upper trapezius triggerband) Common triggerband of the upper back and neck that has a pathway that originates on the top of the shoulder and follows the upper trapezius muscle to the ipsilateral mastoid.

Slide Clunk: Sensation experienced by the patient when a tectonic fixation is corrected.

Slinky Analogy: Metaphor comparing a cylinder distortion to a Slinky® toy in which the coils have become tangled.

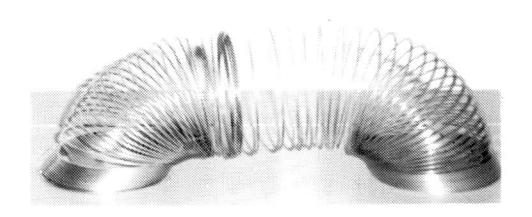

Slipping Rib Syndrome: Folding distortion of the intercostal membrane which forces a rib to intermittently overlap the rib below it.

Slow Tectonic Pump: Exaggerated and deliberate flexing and extending, or abducting and adducting, or tractioning and compressing of limb or other body part to increase synovial fluid circulation in a fixated joint.

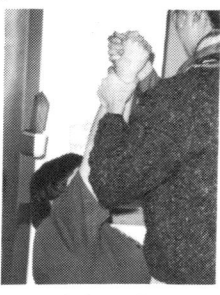

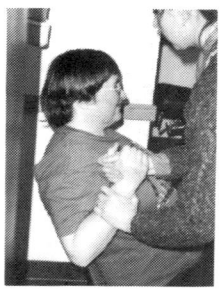

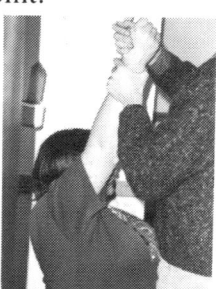

Spasm: Muscular activity from simultaneous but intermittent electrical stimulation of both flexors and extensors.

Speed: Amount of time it takes for an extremity to complete its motion. A grading scale of one to four quantifies this ability.

Sprain: Unspecified fascial distortion of a joint.

Squeegee Cylinder Technique: Form of cylinder technique in which the physician's hands wrap around a portion of the affected extremity and with a squeezing motion slide smoothly along the limb. Note squeegee can also be utilized to treat broad areas of tangled cylinder fascia on the trunk.

Staccato Manipulation: Series of small clicks felt or heard as a folding distortion is corrected with folding technique.

Star Folding Distortion: Folding distortion located between the ribs and beneath the star triggerband starting point. It is treated by first correcting the star triggerband (if present) followed by traction/thrust of the intercostal membrane.

Star Triggerband: Most common and most prominent triggerband of the thoracic area. It has a course that begins halfway between the shoulder blade and the spine in the mid-scapular area. It is treated by ironing out the triggerband from the starting point upward to either the ipsilateral or contralateral mastoid process. Star triggerbands often are palpated as knots.

Starting Point: Origin of a triggerband pathway and the usual location to begin triggerband technique. Starting points are typically located at the site where crossbands occur.

Stepped Off the Curb Wrong Ankle Sprain: Typical history of a continuum sprained ankle.

Stepped On the Foot Ankle Sprain: Typical history of a folding sprained ankle.

Stepping: Small pathological jerks or hesitations during motion.

Andrew Taylor Still: (1828-1917) American physician who founded osteopathy.

Strain: Unspecified fascial distortion less symptomatic than a sprain.

Strain and Counterstrain Technique: System developed by Lawrence Jones, D.O., FAAO, of relieving musculoskeletal pain. In strain and counterstrain the joint is placed into its position of greatest comfort and the origin and insertion of the associated muscles are approximated to achieve maximum relaxation. In the FDM this is envisioned as relieving the strain by gently forcing the triggerband twist out of the muscle and refolding contorted folding fascia.

Stress Fracture: Abnormality in the density of the bone which occurs when a triggerband is pulled into the bone/ligament transition zone and becomes stuck in the osseous matrix – thus decreasing the density of that portion of the bone.

Stroke: Ischemic event of the brain caused by hemorrhage, thrombosis, or embolism. Fascial distortions on the outside of a blood vessel are postulated to narrow the lumen and disrupt the intima, thereby decreasing the vessel's diameter (and thus blood flow), and increasing turbulence (and the risk of clots forming and dislodging). Also in the FDM the spastic paralysis following a stroke is considered to be the cumulative result of uncorrected fascial distortions within and around muscles that spill and scramble electrical impulses between muscle groups.

Sub-Bands: Individual fibers of a fascial band, ligament, tendon, or other banded fascial structure.

Supraclavicular Herniated Triggerpoint: Large herniated triggerpoint located between the clavicle and the superior margin of the scapula. The SCHTP is often irregularly shaped and protruding portions may occur either medially (i.e., next to the cervical vertebrae) or more laterally. Both medial and lateral protrusions may be present in the same individual.

Tectonic Fixation: Principal type of fascial distortion in which the fascial surface has lost its ability to glide.

Tectonic Technique: Manual method for correcting tectonic fixations by physically forcing the fascial surfaces to slide. Frogleg and reverse frogleg manipulations of the shoulder and hip are examples of tectonic techniques. Non-manipulative tectonic treatments also exist and include the plunger technique, cupping, and steroid injections of joints. Future injection treatments are likely to involve flushing the joint with a synthetic solution, or trans-injecting synovial fluid from a different joint.

Tendonitis: Triggerband, or less commonly a continuum distortion, present in a tendon.

Tennis Elbow/Little Leaguer's Elbow: Tender area over the lateral or medial epicondyle that is caused by either a triggerband or a continuum distortion.

Total Height: Highest vertebral level the fingers can reach during internal rotation of the shoulder.

Traction: Treatment modality in which a pulling force is applied to an injured area of the body. Unfolding distortions may respond to this treatment.

Traction/Thrust: Manipulation in which a sustained pulling force is combined with a rapid pulling or rotational force (HVLA) to unfold folding fascia.

Transition Zone: Intermediate area between two tissue types that contains characteristics of both tissue types. Of particular interest in the FDM is the transition zone between bone and ligament.

Janet Travell: American physician who has stressed the importance of myofascial triggerpoints as a source of pain.

Tremor: Intermittent muscular activity caused by alternating spilling of electricity back and forth between flexors and extensors.

Triggerband: Principal fascial distortion type characterized as a distorted fascial band.

Triggerband Pathway: Anatomical course that a distorted fascial band is found to have during its correction with triggerband technique. Patients with the same symptoms tend to have the same anatomical pathways.

Triggerband Technique: Manual approach to treating distorted fascial bands in which the distortion is located and corrected along its entire pathway by physical force from the physician's thumb. During triggerband technique the distorted fascial band is untwisted and the separated fibers are forced back together. In chronic pain the adhesions are intentionally fractured with the treatment.

Triggerband Thumb: Sore and swollen treating thumb from attempting too many triggerband corrections before strength and stamina have developed. The underlying injury is a refolding distortion.

Triggerpoint: An undifferentiated fascial distortion. Upon palpation triggerpoints can be categorized into principal fascial distortion types. Those that can be induced to move during treatment are triggerbands (the triggerpoint is in fact the starting point for triggerband technique), those that are found at the junction of ligament or tendon with bone are continuum distortions, and those that protrude above the fascial plane are herniated triggerpoints.

Tripped Down the Stairs Ankle Sprain: Typical history of a triggerband sprained ankle.

Turtle Position: Refolding maneuver of the thoracic spine.

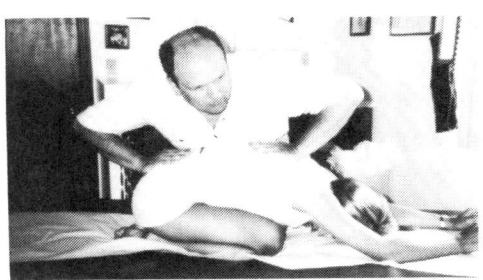

Twist: Triggerband subtype that occurs when a portion of the fascial band becomes rotated on itself.

Twisted Shoulder Harness Analogy: Comparison made between a triggerband and a car shoulder harness to illustrate that a twisted fascial band becomes caught in the belly of the muscle in a similar manner as a twisted shoulder harness belt becomes caught in its harness holder.

Unfolding Distortion: Subtype of folding distortion in which the fascia has unfolded contorted, and can't refold completely. Unfolding injuries hurt deep in the joint, feel better with traction and worse with compression, and are treated with traction and/or traction/thrust manipulations (i.e., unfolding techniques).

Unloaded Ligamental Fibers: Uninjured ligamental fibers in the resting or wavy configuration.

Unwinding: Treatment to relieve myofascial restrictions using traction combined with twisting, bending, and compression maneuvers. In unwinding of the extremities the limb may be used as a long lever to follow tight and loose inherent tissue movements. In the FDM, unwinding unfolds or refolds folding fascia and untangles cylinder distortions.

Wall Technique: High-velocity thrusting manipulation of the lower thoracic spine to correct unfolding distortions of the paravertebral fascia. In this procedure the patient is standing and leaning against the wall with palms at shoulder level. The physician applies traction via a double pisiform hand position with the direction of thrust toward the patient's chin.

Wave: Triggerband subtype that is palpated as a wrinkle in the fascia.

Wavy Floor Phenomenon: Experience following dismount from ball therapy in which the floor no longer feels flat.

Whiplash Injury: Condition resulting from a sudden introduction of flexion or extension into the cervical spine. The fascial distortions typically responsible for neck pain and loss of motion are triggerbands, folding distortions, supraclavicular herniated triggerpoints, and continuum distortions.

Whip Technique: Method of treating unfolding distortions and tectonic fixations of the shoulder by repetitively forcing the elbow from flexion to extension.

Wry Neck: Acute restriction of the sternocleidomastoid muscle secondary to a triggerband.

Zip Lock Analogy: Comparison of a triggerband to a Ziploc® bag to emphasize that both have fibers which separate but can be manually re-approximated without any appreciable loss of function.

INDEX

A

Abdominal herniated triggerpoint, 16, 25, 28, 139-140, 195-196, 207, 215

Abdominal pain, 16, 28, 139-140, 195-196, 215

Abdominal triggerband, 28, 140, 207

Achilles tendon (calcaneal tendon), 7, 65

Acromioclavicular sprain (separated shoulder), 94, 96-98, 129-130, 156

Acupressure, 24

Acupuncture, 221

Adhesions, 21, 24, 37, 39, 50-51, 59, 66-68, 78, 82, 88, 100-101, 154, 158-159, 164, 166, 176-177, 182, 212, 221, 224-226, 229, 231, 235, 238

Adhesive capsulitis, 53, 215, 221

All-or-none principle, 33, 164, 221

Allopathic medicine, 221

Anatomical continuum, 9

Aneurysm, 28, 72, 221

Angina, 221

Ankle eversion, 113, 221

Ankle fracture, 10-11, 37, 114, 123, 153-154, 181

Ankle sprain, 3-4, 13, 16, 29, 32, 34, 37, 63, 111-126, 143, 154, 169-170, 181-182, 193-194, 210, 215, 218, 221-222, 224, 230, 236-237, 239

Anterior ankle continuum distortion (AACD), 114-120, 122-125, 170, 213, 222

Anterior shoulder pathway, 22-23, 53, 90, 92, 95, 99, 103, 106, 130, 147, 174, 178, 202, 222

Aponeuroses, 6, 23

Arteriosclerosis, 72, 222

Asthma, 72, 185, 187-188, 222, 234

B

Ball therapy, 43, 166, 190, 222, 230, 239

Banded herniated triggerpoint, 214, 217, 222

Behind-the-eye headache, 127-128, 201, 223, 230

Biliary colic (gall bladder attack), 16, 28, 139, 196, 223

Bleeding disorder, 28, 44, 72

Body language, 3, 5, 7, 10, 17, 22, 25, 29, 45, 56, 79, 82-83, 85-87, 89-91, 98-99, 112, 125, 127, 134-137, 142, 154-156, 159, 161-166, 169, 179, 181-182, 201-212, 223

Bony triggerband, 59

Bruising, 67-68, 71, 103, 140

Brute force maneuvers, 55, 70, 110, 223

Bull's-eye HTP, 25, 27, 83-84, 86, 140, 157-158, 177, 207-208, 223

Bursitis, 223

Button slipping into the buttonhole analogy, 32, 116, 223

C

Cable ligament, 223

Cancer, 72, 103, 195

Carpal tunnel syndrome, 15, 45, 59, 132-133, 165, 183, 192, 203, 213, 215, 223

Cellulitis, 72, 143

Cervical strain *(also see* Neck pain*)*, 29, 39-40, 75-81, 134

Chair technique, 41-42, 80, 83, 85, 135, 157, 159, 166, 190, 205-207, 223

Chest wall strain, 136-137, 175-176

Collagen vascular disease, 72

Comb technique, 24, 50, 68, 71, 147, 206, 224, 229

Combination distortion, 212, 223-224

Combination sprained ankle, 125, 224

Compression cylinder variant (CCV), 48, 50, 78, 85, 97-98, 100, 141, 213, 224, 226

Compression/thrust, 35, 37-39, 100, 104, 125, 129, 131, 133, 142, 147, 149, 174, 194, 205, 207-208, 210, 219, 224, 227, 234

Connective tissue highway, 10

Continuum distortion, 4, 10-11, 13-16, 29-34, 58-59, 62-63, 69, 75, 77, 79, 80, 82-84, 87, 90, 92, 94-99, 102, 104, 113-120, 122-125, 128-133, 135-137, 141-144, 157, 164, 170, 174, 176-178, 192-193,

206, 212-214, 218, 222-227, 229-230, 232-235, 238, 240

Continuum model of anatomy, 224

Continuum sprained ankle, 16, 32, 63, 111-114, 117-121, 125-126, 143, 169-170, 210, 215, 221, 236

Continuum technique, 13, 16, 29-30, 32-34, 63, 68-69, 71, 77, 80, 83-84, 94-95, 97, 102, 107, 113-114, 116-122, 129, 132-133, 135, 140, 143-144, 157, 164, 176-177, 191, 201-211, 213, 218, 221, 225, 231, 235

Contraindications to FDM techniques, 28, 44, 71-72, 134

Contusion, 132, 165, 215, 218, 225

Cornstarch/water phenomenon, 9, 225

Cortisone injection (*also see* Steriod), 171, 225

Costochondritis, 175, 225

Cows through the barn door analogy, 27, 225

Cranial technique, 128, 201, 225

Crisscrossing fascial bands, 225

Crossband, 21-23, 221, 225, 236

Crosslink, 20-21, 63-67, 82, 221, 225

Crumple, 6, 145, 178, 214, 216, 225

Cupping, 55-56, 71, 102, 226, 237

Cylinder distortion, 4, 13-16, 24, 45-46, 48, 50, 58-59, 68-70, 75, 78-79, 81-82, 85, 90, 92, 96-98, 100, 104, 125-126, 130-133, 141-144, 148, 156-157, 166, 172, 176-179, 185-186, 192-194, 198, 206, 212-214, 220, 223, 225-227, 231, 233-235, 239, 249

Cylinder fascia, 45, 48-50, 72, 132, 166, 172, 220, 224, 226, 231, 236

Cylinder shuffle, 143, 226

Cylinder sprained ankle, 16, 125-126, 210

Cylinder technique, 45-50, 68-70, 78, 81, 83, 85, 97-100, 102, 104-105, 109, 117, 125, 128, 131, 133, 140-143, 156-157, 166, 172, 177-178, 186, 193-194, 198, 201-211, 213, 215, 220, 224, 226, 229-230, 236

D

Dislocation, 37, 59, 94, 96-98, 104, 134, 156, 174, 215

Distorted fascial band (*also see* Triggerband), 5-7, 9, 13, 17, 20-21, 59, 76, 79, 214, 216, 221, 225, 234, 238

Dog technique (*see* Kirksville crunch), 52, 81, 159, 206

Double pisiform thrust, 57, 81

Double thumb cylinder technique, 47-50, 68-69, 78, 81, 83, 85, 91, 98, 100, 109, 125, 128, 140-141, 143-144, 166, 186, 193-194, 198, 201-203, 205-210, 220, 224, 226

Double twist, 226, 229

E

Ear pain, 129

Edema, 72, 143

Elbow pain, 15, 130-131, 191, 203

Epicondylitis, 130, 191-192

Erythema, 71, 197

Everted continuum distortion, 4, 30-31, 33, 84, 118, 193, 213-214, 218, 226, 233

External rotation of shoulder, 92-95, 99, 103, 155-156, 171, 173-176, 185, 187, 197, 226

F

Facet tectonic fixation, 51, 53, 57, 75, 77-79, 81, 100, 102, 104, 135, 224

Fascial band, 3, 5-9, 12-13, 17-18, 20-23, 59, 68, 72, 76, 79, 82, 128, 130, 178, 185, 214, 216, 221-223, 225-226, 229-231, 234, 237-239

Fascial distortion model (FDM), 3-7, 9-10, 13, 21, 24, 29, 31, 35, 45, 62-63, 65-69, 71, 81, 88, 96, 98, 125, 127, 130, 132, 137-139, 141, 145-146, 159, 166, 180, 184, 186, 190, 192, 198, 213, 221-223, 225, 227, 231-233, 237-239, 249

Fascial fiber, 5-9, 12-13, 20-21, 59, 63, 75-76, 78, 82, 101, 127, 135-136, 143, 178, 180, 185-186, 221, 224-227, 233-234

Fascial fluid transport system, 10-11, 62-63, 154, 170

Fascial plane, 14, 25-28, 35, 37, 69, 76, 84, 127, 178, 180, 214, 217, 222, 227, 229, 231, 238

Fasciitis, 144, 163-164, 210, 227, 229, 233

Fibromyalgia, 15, 24, 82, 167-168, 183, 206, 222, 227

Finger sprain, 15, 133-134, 204, 215

First-rib folding distortion, 79-81, 102, 104, 168, 206

Flail chest, 136, 137

Flank herniated triggerpoint, 137-138, 207, 227
Flank triggerband, 137-138, 207, 227
Flaring, 93, 197, 227
Floppy leg phenomena, 183
Fluidity, 103, 227
Folding distortion, 3-4, 10-11, 13-16, 35-44, 58-61, 67, 70, 75, 77, 79-83, 85-88, 90-92, 94-97, 100, 102, 104, 114, 121, 123, 125, 131-133, 135, 143, 146-149, 154, 157-160, 162, 166, 168, 174, 176-177, 179, 182, 198, 206, 212-214, 219, 222, 227, 229-231, 234-236, 239-240
Folding fascia, 4, 14, 36-37, 39, 45, 57, 70, 82, 143, 156, 194, 219, 224, 227, 235, 237-239
Folding/high-velocity manipulation, 227
Folding sprained ankle, 5, 13, 16, 112-114, 117, 123-125, 143, 150-154, 181-182, 210, 215, 221, 237
Folding technique, 13, 35, 39, 43, 57, 59, 68, 70, 77, 85, 94-95, 102, 104, 108, 113, 117, 123, 140, 143, 157, 159, 162, 176, 182, 198, 203-204, 207, 209-211, 213, 215, 222, 227, 230, 236
Folding/thrusting, 40, 43, 70, 130, 147, 176, 223, 227
Foot inversion, 227
Foot sprain, 16, 125, 143-144, 169-170, 210, 215, 227
Forearm cross, 228
Forearm pain, 131-132, 203
Fracture, 10-11, 29, 37, 45, 59, 60-61, 70, 72, 94, 96-98, 103, 114, 119, 122-124, 126-127, 130-132, 134, 136, 143-144, 153-154, 156, 165-166, 181, 193-194, 204, 210-211, 215, 218, 221, 228, 237
Frogleg tectonic manipulation, 51, 53-57, 70, 83, 85, 87, 101, 110, 131, 140, 158-159, 186, 191, 202-203, 206, 208-210, 228, 237
Frozen shoulder, 3-5, 13, 62, 89, 98, 101-103, 130, 147, 156, 183, 185, 187, 215, 228

G

Gall bladder attack (cholecystitis, *see* Biliary colic)
Gerlach, U.J., 12
Global loss of motion of shoulder, 53, 94-98, 101-102, 130, 156, 166, 178, 228,
Godman, John, 228
Grain of salt, 128, 214, 216, 228

Groin strain, 16, 141, 228

H

Hallelujah maneuver, 39, 41, 80, 104, 135, 166, 168, 206, 228
Hand direction, 93, 103, 175-176, 228
Hand pain, 133, 197-198, 204
Hand rotation, 66, 93, 96, 103-104, 228
Headache, 25, 127-128, 201, 223, 230
Headlight effect, 226, 228
Heart attack (*also see* Myocardial infarction), 72
Heat, 34, 58, 71-72, 98, 101, 103-104, 119, 126, 131, 134-135, 140, 147, 171, 187, 194
Heel spur continuum distortion, 144, 229
Hematoma, 72
Herniated triggerpoint (HTP), 13-16, 25-28, 69, 83-84, 86, 94-95, 128, 137-140, 158, 201, 207, 212-214, 217, 221-223, 227, 229-231, 235
Herniated triggerpoint therapy, 25-28, 68-69, 71, 83, 86, 94-95, 99, 101-102, 127-128, 138-140, 157, 195-196, 198, 202, 205, 207-208, 213, 229
Hesitation, 229
High-velocity low-amplitude osteopathic manipulation (HVLA), 4, 33, 42, 77-78, 80, 100, 102, 104, 134-135, 213, 218, 224, 229, 231, 238
Hip pain, 16, 208
Hit-by-truck effect, 72, 229
Hylan G-F 20, 62
Hypertension, 44, 72, 195
Hypertonicity, 5, 145, 229

I

Ice, 3, 31, 34, 71-72, 96, 98, 103-104, 118-119, 122, 124, 128, 130, 132, 134-135, 140-141, 171-172, 175, 187, 193
Ice/slush/water analogy, 31, 229
Iliotibial tract, 84, 86, 148, 177-178
Impingement syndrome, 89, 173
Indian burn cylinder technique, 48-50, 68, 70, 98, 104, 125, 131, 133, 141-143, 192, 194, 198, 203-204, 206, 208-209, 211, 224, 226, 229

Inflammation, 10-11, 89, 231
Integrated neuromusculoskeletal release (INR), 229
Interosseous membrane, 10-11, 37, 59-61, 70, 132, 143, 145, 147, 149, 154, 178, 203
Interseptal membrane, 192
Inversion therapy, 39, 42-44, 85, 157, 159, 166, 190, 206, 230
Inverted continuum distortion, 30-31, 33, 77, 84, 193, 213-214, 218, 224, 229-230, 233, 235

J

Jones, Lawrence, 237
Jumping, 13-14, 45, 47, 69, 126, 192, 215, 230

K

Karate-chop hand arrangement, 230
Key bronchus triggerband, 230
Kidney stone pain (*also see* Renal colic), 16, 137-139, 207, 215
Kirksville crunch (*also see* Dog technique), 51, 57, 81, 104, 158-159, 168, 206
Knee sprain, 16, 37-39, 141-142
Knot, 141, 214, 216, 230, 233, 236

L

Lacrimal herniated triggerpoint, 128, 201, 223, 230
Lateral ankle continuum distortion, 10, 32, 118-119, 125, 170
Lateral ankle triggerband pathway, 114, 121-122, 230
Lateral collateral ligament of knee, 9
Lateral recumbent folding technique, 230
Lateral thigh triggerband (iliotibial band triggerband), 83-84, 86, 157, 208
Leg pain, 142-143, 209
Lierse, W., 12
Ligament, 3, 6, 9, 13-14, 17, 29-33, 59, 62-65, 77, 111, 114, 116, 118-119, 122, 135, 143-144, 178, 189, 215, 218, 223-226, 229-231, 233, 235, 237, 239
Ligamental/tendon tear, 65
Ligamental triggerband, 59, 63, 64

Loaded ligamental fibers, 64, 231
Low back pain (lumbar strain), 4, 15, 27, 37, 39, 42, 56, 75, 82-88, 140, 157-159, 165, 183, 189, 207-208, 213, 231
Low back pain with thigh tightness triggerband (posterior thigh tightness triggerband), 82-83, 86, 140, 157-158, 207, 231
Lumbar roll, 57, 206
Lunging, 231

M

Massage, 24, 231
McBurney's point, 28, 231
Mechanical sensory system, fascia as, 8, 10, 185, 222
Milking, 25-26, 69, 231
Mixing, 24
Movement, 24, 75, 121, 215, 231
Muscle energy technique, 177, 231
Myocardial infarction, 231, 249
Myofascial release technique, 24, 229, 231
Myofascial triggerpoint, 231, 238

N

Neck pain (*also see* Cervical strain), 15, 25, 76, 134, 204-205, 215, 240
Neutral thrust, 57, 77-78, 81, 104, 201, 205-207, 224, 231
Non-banded herniated triggerpoint, 217, 231

O

Orthopathic medicine, 3-4, 16, 68, 213, 232, 249
Orthopathy, 3-5, 147, 232
Osteoarthritis, 63, 72, 161-162, 189, 204, 232
Osteomyelitis, 72
Osteopathic medicine, 232,
Osteopathy, 4, 232, 237,
Osteoporosis, 44, 63, 72, 134, 233
Overshift, 30-31, 33, 233
Overuse syndrome, 158, 160

P

Pancreatitis, 28, 139, 196
Paresthesias, 46
Pea, 214, 216, 233
Pelvic pain, 28, 139
Percussion hammer, 233
Periscapular triggerband, 102, 104, 135
Petechiae, 56, 71
Phlebitis, 71-72
Physiological continuum, 9, 185
Pitch, 8, 233
Plantar fasciitis, 144, 163-164, 210, 227, 229, 233
Plunger technique, 51, 55, 71, 101, 147, 158, 233, 237
Posterior shoulder pathway, 53, 79-80, 91-92, 95, 99, 103-104, 106, 147, 168, 174, 178, 202, 206, 233
Post-polio syndrome, 183-184
Post-stroke spastic paralysis (PSSP), 4-5, 143, 145-150, 177-178, 213
Pregnancy, 72
Pressure points, 233
Principal types of fascial distortions, 13, 100, 214-215, 224, 226-227, 229, 234, 237-238
Prone tectonic technique of shoulder, 101, 147, 234
Pseudo-sciatica, 234
Psoriatic arthritis, 197-198
Pulled muscle, 5-7, 13, 66, 208, 215, 234
Purse string effect, 222, 230, 234

Q

Quick victory strategy, 116, 234

R

Refolding distortion, 35, 37-39, 42, 51, 77, 79, 81, 90, 102, 104, 128-129, 143-144, 166, 193-194, 212-214, 219, 233-234, 238
Registered Orthopathist, 249
Release, 25-28, 32, 34, 37, 49, 69, 77-78, 80, 84-85, 116, 118-119, 123, 125, 129, 132, 136, 138-139, 142, 144, 164, 225, 231, 234-235
Reflex sympathetic dystrophy, 45, 185-186
Renal colic (flank pain, *also see* Kidney stone pain), 16, 25, 72, 137-139, 207, 215, 235
Retinaculum, 3, 6, 22, 59, 132, 203, 223, 226
Reverse frogleg tectonic manipulation, 51, 53-57, 70, 85, 87, 101, 110, 131, 140, 147-149, 158-159, 186, 191, 202-203, 206, 208-210, 228, 237
Rib injuries, 15, 136-137
Roadblock effect, 62-63, 185
Road map analogy, 60-61, 235
Rolfing, 24, 235
Rotator cuff injuries, 89
Ruptured quadriceps tendon, 59
Ruptured viscus, 28

S

Sacroiliac strain, 29, 84-85, 215, 218
SCHTP, *see* Supraclavicular herniated triggerpoint
Scissors technique, 83-84, 140, 207, 235
Sclerotherapy, 235
Separated shoulder, *see* Acromioclavicular sprain
Shifting of the continuum, 9, 30, 235
Shin splints, 16, 142, 209
Shoulder to mastoid triggerband, *see* Upper trapezius triggerband
Slide clunk, 55, 57, 235
Slinky analogy, 14, 48, 235
Slipping rib syndrome, 136, 236
Slow tectonic pump, 51, 53-57, 101, 147, 158-159, 186, 188, 202, 236
Sodium Hyaluronate, 62
Sore shoulder, 4, 14, 22, 24-25, 29, 37, 66, 75-76, 79-80, 89-90, 92-96, 98-103, 130, 147, 156, 166, 178, 215
Spasm, 5, 45-46, 75, 78-79, 81, 83, 85, 92, 128, 134, 145-148, 177, 215, 223, 235-236
Speed, 11, 66, 93, 103, 115, 173-176, 183, 185, 197, 231, 236
Spinal stenosis, 189-190
Splint, 6, 11, 16, 67, 111, 117, 119, 122, 124-126
Sprained ankle, *see* Ankle sprain
Squeegee cylinder technique, 48-50, 68, 70, 78, 81, 85, 98, 109, 141, 143, 186, 194, 202-203, 206, 208-209, 224, 226, 236

Staccato manipulation, 37, 236
Standing lift, *see* Hallelujah maneuver
Star folding distortion, 53, 79-81, 100, 104, 136, 168, 205-206, 236
Star triggerband, 53, 75-76, 79-81, 90, 92, 100-104, 106, 127, 135, 168, 179-180, 204-206, 216, 236
Starting point, 21-24, 75, 79-80, 84, 99, 104, 114, 120-122, 130, 136, 164, 168, 213, 222, 233, 236, 238
Stepped off the curb wrong ankle sprain, 111-113, 236
Stepped on the foot ankle sprain, 112-113, 237
Stepping, 93, 169, 175-176, 185, 237
Steroid *also see* Cortisone injection, 4, 62-63, 89, 237
Still, Andrew Taylor, 232, 237
Strain, 4, 25, 29, 42, 45, 66, 75-81, 85, 130, 134-137, 141, 175, 179, 218, 237
Strain and counterstrain technique, 237
Stress fracture, 63, 194, 237
Stroke, 4-5, 71-72, 143, 145-150, 177, 184, 213, 237, 249
Sub-bands, 8, 17, 21-22, 237
Supraclavicular herniated triggerpoint (SCHTP), 25-27, 53, 75-76, 79-80, 82, 90, 92, 95-97, 99-104, 107, 127, 130, 147, 168, 174, 177-180, 186, 198, 202, 205-206, 213, 237, 240
Synovial fluid, 14, 51-55, 62, 102, 154, 178, 184, 186, 188, 223, 225, 236-237

T

Tectonic fixation, 4, 13-16, 37, 51-53, 55-59, 62, 67, 70, 72, 75, 77-79, 81-83, 85, 87, 91-92, 95-96, 98, 100-102, 104, 128-129, 131, 135, 148, 149, 154, 157-159, 164, 177-178, 183-188, 192-193, 206, 212-214, 221, 224, 226, 228-230, 233-235, 237, 240
Tectonic technique, 37, 51-58, 68, 70-71, 83, 87, 95, 101-102, 104, 110, 140, 147-148, 157-159, 183-184, 186, 188, 191, 201, 203-204, 208-210, 213, 215, 222-223, 228, 231, 234, 237
Temporomandibular joint (TMJ), 128-129, 201, 213
Tendon, 3, 6-7, 13, 17, 29, 59, 62, 65, 89, 131-132, 144, 178, 215, 218, 224, 226, 229, 233, 237-238
Tendonitis, 7, 62, 89, 131-132, 215, 222, 238
Tennis elbow, 14, 130, 238

Thigh pain, 141, 208, 231
Thoracic strain (upper back pain), 15, 79-81, 135, 179, 205-206
Thrusting manipulation *(also see* High-velocity low-amplitude osteopathic manipulation), 4, 31, 34, 40, 42-43, 67, 70, 84, 105, 129-130, 135, 140, 147, 176, 222-223, 227, 239
Thumb sprain, 133
Thumb techniques, 68-70
Toe fracture, 144, 211
Toe sprain, 144, 211
Total height, 66, 93, 103, 175-176, 197-198, 238
Traction, 3, 14, 27, 35-45, 48-50, 53, 55, 57, 61, 70, 77-78, 80-81, 85, 97, 104, 121, 123-124, 126, 129, 131-133, 135, 141-144, 148, 157, 159, 162, 166, 190, 192, 219-220, 222-223, 226-227, 229-231, 234, 236, 238-239
Traction/thrust, 35, 37-39, 40-42, 70, 80, 85, 100, 104, 117, 121-122, 124, 129, 131, 133-134, 142, 147, 149, 198, 201-202, 205, 207-208, 210, 227, 230, 236, 238-239
Transition zone, 9, 13-14, 29-33, 59, 62-63, 69, 77, 80, 84, 98, 116, 118, 131, 164, 178, 213-214, 218, 221, 224-226, 229-230, 233, 235, 237-238
Travell, Janet, 238
Tremor, 5, 145-146, 238
Triggerband, 4-7, 10-24, 28, 34, 37, 39, 50, 52-53, 56, 58-59, 62-67, 69, 75-76, 78-79, 82-83, 85-86, 92, 94-95, 97-101, 104-106, 111, 113-114, 120-122, 125, 127-144, 148, 154, 158-159, 164, 166, 170, 176-178, 182, 185-186, 192-193, 206, 212-214, 216-217, 221-231, 233-240, 249
Triggerband sore shoulder, 22, 24, 89
Triggerband sprained ankle, 13, 16, 63, 111-114, 117, 121-122, 143, 210, 215, 221, 230, 239
Triggerband technique, 7, 13, 16-17, 19-24, 28, 34, 37, 56, 59, 64-65, 67-69, 71-72, 75-76, 78-79, 83, 86, 88-89, 94-95, 97, 99, 101-102, 113, 117, 120-121, 127-129, 131, 133, 135-136, 138-141, 143, 147-148, 157, 164, 166, 171, 176, 182, 193, 201-205, 207-211, 213, 215-217, 225, 229-231, 236, 238
Triggerband thumb, 133, 238
Triggerpoint, 231, 238
Tripped down the stairs ankle sprain, 111-113, 239

Turtle position, 206, 239
Twist, 6-7, 13, 17-19, 24, 62-63, 65, 75, 82, 120, 127-128, 133, 136, 214, 216, 222, 225-226, 229, 231, 233, 237, 239
Twisted shoulder harness analogy, 24, 239

U

Unfolding distortion, 14, 35-42, 55, 60, 77, 80, 85, 91, 100, 104, 112, 128-129, 131-135, 142, 148, 160, 166, 172, 182, 193, 213-214, 219, 238-240
Unloaded ligamental fibers, 64, 239
Unwinding, 239
Upper arm pain, 46, 92, 94-96, 98, 105, 130, 155-156, 165, 171, 202-203, 215
Upper trapezius triggerband (shoulder to mastoid triggerband), 75-76, 79, 91-92, 96, 101-103, 106, 127, 147, 168, 204-206, 235

V

Vasovagal response, 72, 97

W

Wall technique, 41, 80, 157, 159, 168, 206, 239
Wave, 64-65, 214, 216, 239
Wavy floor phenomenon, 239
Whiplash injury, 77, 127, 240
Whip technique, 37, 55, 102, 108, 110, 133, 158-159, 240
Whole hand techniques, 68, 70
Wrist pain, 132-133
Wry neck, 134-135, 204, 240

Z

Zip lock analogy, 17-20, 121, 240

About the Author

STEPHEN TYPALDOS, D.O.

Originator of the fascial distortion model and techniques, Dr. Typaldos specializes in the manipulative treatment of athletic and non-athletic extremity injuries. He is a 1986 graduate of the University of Health Sciences College of Osteopathic Medicine in Kansas City, Missouri, and completed a rotating internship at Parkview Hospital (Osteopathic) and a family practice residency at Mercy Hospital, both in Toledo, Ohio. For more than five years he practiced emergency medicine in which the orthopathic approach to acute injuries was developed and refined. Dr. Typaldos' office, the Osteopathic Extremity Clinic, is in Brewer, Maine.

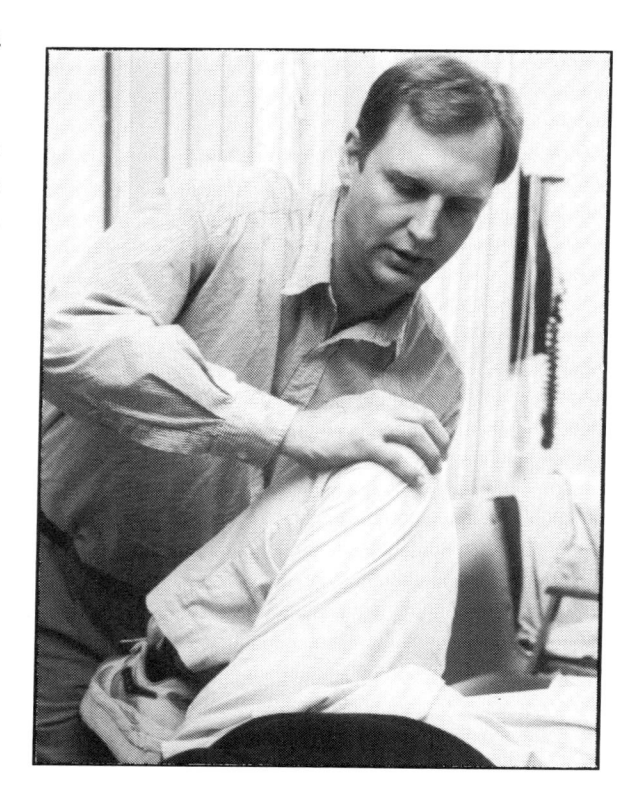

Author's Postscript Note

As the spring flowers bloom across New England, this third edition of *Orthopathic Medicine: The Unification of Orthopedics with Osteopathy Through the Fascial Distortion Model* makes its debut. Along with its German and French language counterparts (also soon to be published), this text has been specifically designed to lead the practitioner through the clinical and theoretical aspects of orthopathy. In particular, the case history section has been added to show not only the breadth and depth of orthopathic medicine, but that medical problems of a wide variety can be contemplated through the fascial distortion model.

Currently, orthopathic practitioners consist of two groups of individuals: 1. American physicians (M.D.'s and D.O.'s), and 2. International osteopaths (some of whom are also M.D.'s). However, in the near future I expect physicians not just to focus on the clinical manipulative branch of orthopathy (which is mostly presented in this book) but to contribute to the building of orthopathic medicine itself by:

- Improving orthopedic surgical procedures
- Adding FDM concepts to radiological interpretations
- Initiating new FDM strategies in the practice of internal medicine

The current training of orthopathists involves three levels of seminars which are available in Europe, Japan, Canada, and the United States. Note that:

- Physicians or international osteopaths who take all three levels of the seminars, pass written and practical exams, and submit a thesis of acceptable quality on any of the clinical or basic science aspects of orthopathy, will be eligible to become a *Registered Orthopathist*.

Although this book lays the groundwork for the current practice of orthopathy, it only touches the surface of the medical possibilities. Perhaps by the end of the next decade partially paralyzed stroke patients will recover within weeks, and orthopedics will be revolutionized through the development of intrasurgical FDM techniques. And perhaps even myocardial infarctions will be prevented by endoscopic laser obliterations of coronary artery triggerbands and cylinder distortions. These are the medical challenges of the 21st century in which the fascial distortion model seeks to be the bridge between incremental advancements and exponential leaps.

Stephen Typaldos, D.O.
April 1999

ORTHOPATHIC GLOBAL HEALTH PUBLICATIONS
c/o Osteopathic Extremity Clinic
(207) 989-5879
399 South Main Street
Brewer, Maine, 04412
USA